The Lost Secrets of
AYURVEDIC ACUPUNCTURE

AN AYURVEDIC GUIDE TO ACUPUNCTURE

Based upon the Suchi Veda Science of Acupuncture
The Traditional Indian System

by Dr. FRANK ROS A.M.D., D.Ac.
Doctor of Ayurvedic Acupuncture and Medicine

Life Member of Acupuncture Society of India Member of Naturopathic
Practitioners Assoc. Inc.
and Australian Association of Ayurveda
Director of Australian Institute of Ayurvedic Medicine

LOTUS PRESS
Twin Lakes, Wisconsin 53181 U.S.A.

DISCLAIMER

This book is a reference work, not intended to diagnose, prescribe or treat. The information contained herein is in no way to be considered as a substitute for consultation with a professional physician. Proper training under a competent Ayurvedic Acupuncture physician in an appropriate college is essential or most desirable.

FIRST EDITION, 1994
Printed in the United States of America.

ISBN 0-914955-12-8   CIP 93-80314

Library of Congress Cataloging in Publication Data:

Ros, Frank.
    The lost secrets of ayurvedic acupuncture.

Published 1994 by Lotus Press/ P.O. Box 325, Twin Lakes WI 53181 USA

DEDICATION

To my darling wife, Judy
and son, Clinton with much love.

ACKNOWLEDGMENTS

A debt of gratitude to Professor Dr. P.H. Kulkarni, Research Guide (and former Ayurvedic Dean), Poona University (Pune) for his perseverance and support and to my good colleagues, Ayurvedic physicians Professor Manfred Junius F.I.I.M. and Dr. Krishna Kumar, F.I.I.M. for their openness, friendship and understanding. Gurukal Scaife — It was an honor being your student.

CONTENTS

FOREWORD

Ayurveda and Chinese Medicine are the two oldest and best developed of the natural healing traditions of humanity. This is not surprising, as they are the medical systems of India and China, the largest and oldest of the world's civilizations. The two systems have come to the forefront again, with the revival of traditional medicine that is happening today throughout the world. We are recognizing that traditional medicine, like the Earth itself, has special powers of healing, particularly for deep seated disorders, that we have overlooked in the rush to develop a standardized technologically-based medicine. To deal with the problems caused by technology, stress, artificial life-styles and global pollution we are once again seeing the value of these natural healing systems and their ability to harness the very life-force of nature itself.

Both systems, which are recognized by the World Health Organization, are now being practiced, and Chinese medicine itself is becoming legalized, all over the world. The medicine of the coming century is bound to have a powerful imprint from both these two ancient currents of healing, which offer safe and proven remedies as an alternative to the allopathic medicine whose limitations, particularly in the treatment of chronic diseases, are becoming evident everywhere.

Naturally, an attempt to connect these two important systems of medicine is already happening. Students of one system will usually have an interest in the other. Chinese acupuncture itself is now being practiced in India. Ayurvedic medicine is developing in Japan and may perhaps soon be introduced into China as well.

The two systems possess an affinity for language, approach and methodology, with their emphasis on the life-force, the elements and qualities of nature. In Chinese medicine, this takes the form of yin

and yang, chi and the five elements of earth, water, fire, wood and
metal. In Ayurvedic medicine, it takes the form of the three Doshas
or biological humors (Vata, Pitta and Kapha) and the five elements
of earth, water, fire, air and ether. Both systems speak of wind, fire
and phlegm disorders and employ similar methodologies to treat them.
Both systems classify food and herbs by taste, element and heating
or cooling energy.

Both Chinese and Ayurvedic medicine are based upon systems that
are built into the oldest layers of their cultures. The Chinese system
reflects the language of the I Ching, the oldest Chinese book. The
Ayurvedic system reflects the language of the Vedas, the oldest of the
books of India. They are not simply extraneous medical systems practiced by an educated elite but rooted in the entire culture and in the
very life of the common people of their countries. These include the
diet and folk medicines of the various local cultures of their diverse
regions. Such a living system of healing that includes self-healing and
home remedies is exactly what we need today, to reintegrate medicine
into life.

The two systems also have many historical links. India and China
have maintained a steady commerce of trade and exchange of ideas
going back to prehistoric times. Though the two subcontinents are
next to each other, their separation by the high Tibetan plateau, the
Central Asian desert and the jungles of southeast Asia has made contact difficult, but not impossible. The Silk Trail between China and
the West always involved a trade route from China to India. Sea routes
from the South of India to southern China have also been in existence
for over two thousand years. Tibet itself represents a composite culture
of India and Chinese influence which includes both these medical
systems. The most notable contact between India and China was
through the movement of Buddhism from India, but links before and
after these periods existed as well.

In my own studies I became interested in both systems at an early
point. After having examined both systems in depth, it became clear
to me that the differences between the two are more semantic than

substantial, and that by changing a few key terms, the corpus of knowledge of one system can be translated into the other, thus significantly widening the scope of each. However, preoccupation with other pursuits has not left me the time to pursue this matter in detail. Therefore, it is heartening to see other people take up such a pursuit. This volume is an excellent example.

Much of the herbal medicine of the Chinese and Ayurvedic system shows points of commonality. That is why in my books *Ayurvedic Healing* and *The Yoga of Herbs*, mention is made of relevant Chinese herbs and formulas to Ayurvedic conditions. Yet the treatment models of Ayurvedic and Chinese medicine, which have similar energetic languages, are not only connected on the level of herbs but also on the level of acupuncture.

Acupuncture is the most visible, unique and conspicuous feature of Chinese medicine. Many of us in the West tend to identify Chinese medicine with acupuncture, though the system itself is predominately herbal in nature. Ayurvedic medicine does not contain such a clearly visible system of pressure point therapy in its practice today as does acupuncture. Yet it does contain traces of such a system. Ayurvedic books contain classifications of special points, called marmas or "sensitive" points. It describes the body in terms of various channel systems (srotamsi or nadis), much like the meridian systems of Chinese medicine.

Unfortunately, Ayurveda and other Vedic systems in India, have been preserved in family traditions and, as a rule, do not share their secrets openly. This means that the knowledge available about Ayurveda in books—even in the Indic languages of which few have been translated into English—represents only a fraction of what is kept hidden and is the subject only of oral transmission. Such secrets of Ayurvedic acupuncture or pressure point therapy can be found in family traditions in India today.

Dr. Frank Ros, an Ayurvedic practitioner and acupuncturist from Australia, in *The Lost Secrets of Ayurvedic Acupuncture*, introduces an Ayurvedic model for the practice of acupuncture. This model is remarkably like the Chinese model, which may be surprising at first to those who know only Chinese medicine. They will see their own system presented according to a slightly different treatment line. As we look more deeply however, we see that the similarities between the two approaches are based upon a common knowledge and common tradition between the two systems.

Dr. Ros has studied the hidden or lost Ayurvedic traditions in India. Martial arts and massage systems, particularly in South India—from which the Chinese martial arts may have developed, along with the movement of Buddhism from South India to China—reflect an acupuncture-like knowledge of the pressure points on the body. South India has been a repository of ancient knowledge of all types in India. It was the main region of refuge in the subcontinent from the cruel Islamic onslaught of the Middle Ages in which most of the monasteries and temples in North India—including the great universities and libraries of Takshashila and Nalanda—were destroyed.

Dr. Ros' book is extremely readable and very practical. He shows how acupuncture can be easily understood in terms of Ayurvedic medicine. Almost any acupuncturist can use the book to incorporate an Ayurvedic point of view into his or her own practice. Similarly, Ayurvedic students can use the book to incorporate acupuncture in their study and practice of Ayurveda. He has established the main translation of terms between Ayurveda and Traditional Chinese Medicine, which itself is useful in attempts to correlate the two systems on all levels. With such an important ground-breaking work (linking the two systems of medicine), their eventual reintegration is bound to be a matter of time.

Whether Chinese medicine may have an Ayurvedic root is bound to remain a debatable point. The antiquity of both systems and the difficulties in historical interpretation make any statements in this regard tentative. Recent historical evidence is also suggesting much greater antiquity for both these ancient cultures. For example, the rediscovery of the ancient Sarasvati river system and the Mehrgarh site, shows an organic development of civilization in India, going

back to 6500 BC, with a strong Vedic (Aryan) presence from the
earliest era. This gives a much greater antiquity to Vedic culture, of
which Ayurveda is a part, than has been previously thought. In my
book *Gods, Sages and Kings: Vedic Secrets of Ancient Civilization*, I tried
to present some of this information, including a small section show-
ing the probable antiquity of Ayurveda, according to this new model.

Meanwhile the antiquity of ancient Chinese culture is also being
extended backwards. We are being forced to recognize that our ancient ancestors had not only spiritual secrets, but secrets of healing,
and possessed cultures that were much older and more sophisticated
than we have yet realized.

In any event, an alliance of Traditional Chinese Medicine and
Ayurveda is bound to emerge, both in terms of herbs and acupuncture. It will greatly broaden the scope of natural healing throughout
the world and will reintroduce natural healing with a strong clinical
model and a vast clinical experience. In this development, the work
of Dr. Ros and his present book, represents an important breakthrough.
We look forward to additional books from the author, going into
greater detail about the profound connection between acupuncture
and Ayurveda.

Dr. David Frawley O.M.D.
December, 1993
Santa Fe, New Mexico

INTRODUCTION

This book reflects over twenty years of study, practice and research on traditional Indian medicine, yet the concepts outlined herein have been developed and refined over thousands of years. This traditional Indian medical system is referred to as Ayurvedic Medicine or Ayurveda.

Ayurveda means the "Science of Life." It is both a curative and a preventive form of therapy. It is also holistic, since the whole person is diagnosed and treated, not just the particular symptom which is evident. It isn't a matter of "my pain is lessened," but rather "I feel better, I am well"; where "I" refers to the person as a whole and not just the localized symptom.

Ayurvedic medicine is thousands of years old, but it is still as relevant today as it was in ancient times. Although no one can yet be sure when it first originated, it is generally well known and agreed that it was utilized in India more than 5000 years ago.

Yoga and Ayurveda are generally considered to have been practiced in the ancient Indus Valley, an area in India (and modern Pakistan) which receives a great deal of attention through present-day archaeological discoveries. It appears as though the people of this area, of Harappas and Mohenjo Daro, suddenly disappeared, or were quickly swallowed up by waves of incoming invaders related to the Aryan civilization.

The first documentation of these concepts occurred only about 2-3 thousand years ago. Previously, they were mainly taught through word-of-mouth, from generation to generation. Nevertheless, the *Vedas* (ancient Indian texts written about 7000 years ago) do mention Ayurvedic medicine and acupuncture (needle therapy). With the flowering of Buddhism in India in 563 BC, learning centers or universities were encouraged and established—especially by the orders of Emperor Ashoka. Hospitals were built and most of the arts and sciences were taught and practiced, especially at the Indian Buddhist university of Takshashila. Even martial arts were taught in these centers by the Buddhist monks. As the Dharma (or buddhist law) did not allow monks to use weapons even for self-defense, unarmed self-defense was practiced.

As explained in the text *Milindapanha*, unarmed self-defense was taught as part of the Nineteen Arts, which also included Medicine (*Milindapanha I*). The *Milindapanha* is a scripture of questions and answers between the buddhist king Milinda and the superior monk Nagasena.

In this text the king asks the monk:

"If revered Nagasena enemies can be restrained by the use of the fists alone, then what is the good of knives, bows and arrows?"

This excerpt demonstrates the expertise (although of a secretive nature) that the monks must have had in unarmed self-defense, even against weapons. This knowledge was employed when Buddhism began to extend not only throughout India but also to most of the oriental countries.

During their travels, the monks encountered thieves and opponents of their new religion. Their reluctant use of unarmed methods of self-defense must have saved many a monk's life and allowed their doctrine to reach the further-most corners of the Orient. China, for instance, built a special monastery at Shaoshih Peak of Sungshan Mountains (Honan province) to accommodate monks travelling to China from India. This monastery, built in 300 AD was called the Shaolin Temple and later became renowned for its expertise in Buddhism, martial arts and medicine.

"KALARI—A very ancient Indian martial art. It is part of the traditional belief that the style is the same as that brought to China from India by Bodhidharma and taught at the Shaolin temple." [1]

Monks later also entered other countries, such as Korea, Japan and Indonesia. Their forms of healing and self-defense were taught to the new local monks which explains why Ayurvedic concepts can be found in most oriental countries today.

"The medical system which spread with Buddhism, Ayurveda or one of its offshoots is still practiced today in Tibet, Central Asia, Sri Lanka, and in parts of China, Japan, Indochina and Indonesia."[2]

With the gradual decline of Buddhism in India (caused by various factors including increased popularity of Hinduism), Buddhist ideas receded into the background and in some cases remained secret. Ayurveda and other arts and sciences were later banned by the British East India Company. Only very traditional practitioners retained and practiced them under threat of execution if discovered.

After Mahatma Gandhi achieved independence for India during the early part of this century, traditional concepts were once again encouraged to be practiced. Unfortunately, the task of finding reputable practitioners from whom to learn all the concepts of Ayurveda correctly has been a formidable task. Today, more and more knowledge is coming to light as reluctant practitioners share their secret and often family-related heirlooms of medicine and martial arts.

World-renowned Ayurvedic physician Dr. Chandrashekkar Thakkur explains:

"In India today, if every family shared its medical secrets as the Chinese have [been obliged to do by the government], we would probably find methods quite as interesting and as effective as the Chinese ones."[3]

There is a wealth of information waiting to be shared with the West but unfortunately, India has always been reluctant to export its ideas, or has not utilized modern marketing techniques to capitalize on its assets. Traditionally, Indians have been more concerned with transcending time than making a profit out of it.

AYURVEDIC ACUPUNCTURE
Ayurvedic medicine has many different branches, as it is the study of the whole body and life. One of these branches is Ayurvedic

Acupuncture. This can be termed an accessory therapy since it was used in conjunction with other forms to effect healing. It belongs more correctly to the branch of surgery, one of the eight medical disciplines of Ayurveda.

Ayurvedic surgery in ancient India was extremely advanced (India was normally considered the most advanced country in surgery in ancient times). Plastic surgery of the nose was a routine operation during Sushruta's time. Sushruta is the ancient renowned Ayurvedic surgeon. Broken bones were also mended with metal pins in much the same way they are today.

Today there is no doubt that Ayurvedic Acupuncture originated from the practice of using needles in surgery and the knowledge of the pressure points (which was also utilized by the surgeons in India).

Notes:
1. *Dictionary of the Martial Arts*, p. 93.
2. *Ayurvedic Medicine*, p. 26.
3. *Modern Guide To Ear Acupuncture*, p. 190.

The Lost Secrets of
AYURVEDIC
ACUPUNCTURE

CHAPTER I

AYURVEDIC ACUPUNCTURE

HISTORY AND BACKGROUND

Over the last twenty or so years, Acupuncture has made great inroads into Western forms of healing; so much so that even the World Health Organization (W.H.O.) concluded that not only is Acupuncture a true form of therapy, but that it also can cure, or treat more than three hundred different types of diseases (*W.H.O. Chronicle* No.34, 1980). It all started when President Nixon visited mainland China and hence the subsequent interest by the West of all things oriental.

Of course, acupuncture in China had declined over the years as a system and very few practitioners were to be found before the Chinese Revolution. Maotse Tung encouraged the return of traditional therapies to compensate for the lack of Western pharmaceutical medicines when fighting the Nationalists (who were supported by the West). It became evident to the Chinese that natural therapies, although almost extinct, were more than just effective. They were necessary, due to the ban of pharmaceuticals, to defeat the West, or at least give the wounded a fighting chance.

The West has taken to acupuncture in a very big way and normally it is regarded as a Chinese therapy. While it is true that the system currently recognized in the West is of Chinese origin and is the best known and publicized, the reality is that acupuncture has also been practiced by various countries for thousands of years. It is not exclusive to the Chinese.

"There is proof that Acupuncture has been practiced in ancient Egypt, Persia, India, etc."[1]

TRADITIONAL INDIAN ACUPUNCTURE

The people of India, whose Ayurvedic medicine is very akin to Chinese medicine, also practiced Acupuncture. There it was regarded as part of surgical therapy, since instruments similar to the ones used in surgery were utilized. In fact, it is totally possible that the establishment of this therapy is due to a natural progression from surgical procedures and instruments used long ago.

As Jurgen Thorwald explains:

> *"The vast variety of Indian surgical instruments which have come down to us from the first millennium A.D. suggest that surgery had developed to an extraordinary extent in early India. The sutures and needles described in the Sushruta texts of several thousand years earlier looked no different [to those used during the nineteenth and twentieth centuries]. Straight and bent needles of bone and bronze were used."* [2]

Ayurvedic Acupuncture is traditionally termed *BhedanKarma* (meaning "Piercing-Through Therapy"), and is a part of the traditional Indian methods of using pressure-points or marmas. These methods are generically referred to as *Marma Chikitsa* (Treatment of Marmas). There is an undeniable connection between Marma Chikitsa and what is today recognized as acupuncture. Acupuncture means *Acus* = needle and *puncture*.

Dr. S.D. Ojha (Ph.D., M.A., LL.B.,I.A.S.) explains:

> *"This highly developed knowledge of medicine [Ayurveda] received patronage of kings [in India]. Thereafter, the time came when ambassadors went to East Asian countries, including Ceylon and Indonesia. Amongst them were some of the Buddhist monks who preached and practiced the Ayurvedic system of medicine. They developed the Marma Chikitsa and it was recognized as Acupuncture technique of treatment for curing various diseases."* [3]

In Ayurveda, acupuncture is more correctly termed "Needling," where needles (of a special, suitable design) are used to penetrate the skin ("piercing through") at strategic points of the body in order to cause a therapeutic effect. The points are positioned along energy channels which connect with major organs and structures of the body.

The term "needling" was utilized by Charaka, the ancient Ayurvedic master physician, who used it not only in reference to using needles in surgery but also in non-surgical medical problems.

*"If the physician comes across a patient suffering from syncope,
then . . . NEEDLING [acupuncture] and BURNING [moxibustion] . . . are
helpful in bringing about consciousness."* [4]

It is obvious from the previous statement that acupuncture (needling)
was known to Charaka, several thousand years ago, since syncope
is a non-surgical disorder.

Dr. Chandrashekkar Thakkur says:

*"one volume of the Vedas, known as the Suchi Veda, translated as the
'art of piercing with a needle', was written about 3000 years ago and deals
entirely with acupuncture."* [5]

One of the major problems today is the availability of all types of
ancient Ayurvedic texts. Sharma and Dash in the Charaka explain that:

*"Some of the ancient texts on Ayurveda are not yet available. Among the
extant ones, the Charaka, Sushruta and Vagbhata are recognized as the
Great Trio."* [6]

It is hoped that those which are not currently available to Western
scholars, will be soon.

Professor Dr. P.H. Kulkarni, Research Guide at Poona University
(Poona, India) and current Director of the Institute of Indian Medicine
(Pune) states the following about Ayurvedic Acupuncture:

*"The Vedic therapeutic methods in India date back to the prehistoric era.
Many Chinese travellers had come to India and have written extensively about
the local treatment practices. Some of the Indian authors even said that people
learnt Acupuncture from Indian experts at Takshashila University [circa 100
B.C.]. It is also said that Ayurvedic texts consisted of Acupuncture principles
and that [most of these] are lost due to unfavorable circumstances in India."* [7]

Buddhism also utilized acupuncture and Ayurveda, which were
subsequently taught to the Tibetans. The Buddha was reportedly
responsible for writing various texts on Indian medicine, which
today the Tibetan buddhists jealously guard. There are four shastras
or texts written by the Buddha, one of these—the Fourth Shastra

indeed explains that Tibet received acupuncture and medicine from India, as Tibetan Dr. Yeshi Donden, former physician to the Dalai Lama confirms in his book:

> " *The Tibetan system, mainly derived from Indian Buddhist medicine centers around restoring and maintaining balance between the three humors called Wind [Vata], Bile [Pitta] and Phlegm [Kapha]. Experienced Tibetan physicians have used the system for more than a thousand years.*"[8] *and "Last [in the Fourth Shastra] is a section dealing with accessory therapy, these include Moxibustion, Acupuncture, Surgery and so forth.*"[9]

This must definitely be a reference to Indian surgery and acupuncture, since China has had no traditional form of surgery, as dissection of the human body was totally prohibited, due to religious beliefs. The Tibetan text itself is of Indian origin.

Any system of true acupuncture must have various components besides the use of needles in order to be regarded as acupuncture.

VITAL POINTS *(Marmas)*

The needles must be inserted into specific reflex points (marmas) which then cause an internal therapeutic reaction. A system which does not take these points into account is not a true system of acupuncture. Charaka once again enlightens us with regard to these points. In Chapter VII (14) he explains:

> *"Beyond what is described above, [the following] can be ascertained from inference only [can only be deduced]. They are enumerated below:*
> 5. **Marma** *[Vital points in the body].*"[10]

In the South of India, these vital or reflex points are called Adankals and are traditionally used by Adankal therapists. Today at least 365 of these points are to be found, with some being more important than others.

> *"Pressure point therapy is an ancient art of healing which was popular in many eastern countries particularly India, China, Japan and Korea. This traditional type of pressure point therapy has been named Acupressure, finger*

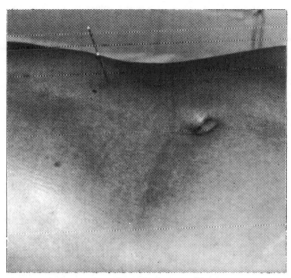

Acupuncture on the abdominal area.

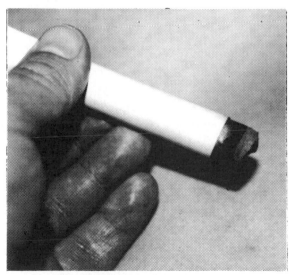

Moxibustion (Agnikarma)

pressure or Adankal therapy." [11]

Sushruta, the ancient renowned Ayurvedic surgeon described these pressure points as being areas of very high concentration of life-energy:

> *"According to Sushruta, every Marma [reflex] point is a seat of Prana [life-energy]. The marmas are similarly located on the body as Acupuncture points."* [12]

Lethal Marmas

There are basically about 107 pressure points considered extremely lethal if a blow to one of these is received. These marmas are the lethal marmas which Sushruta and Charaka both described due to their susceptibility to trauma or injury during battles/wars. An Ayurvedic surgeon was well acquainted with these in case the body was pierced by arrows or spears at one of these locations. The marma's connection with the Ayurvedic concept of the Five Elements would determine whether trauma to one of these points was lethal: either instantly, delayed, or occurring only after the arrow was removed.

Those marmas which are related to the element Fire, would tend to cause instant death since fire can be easily "snuffed out." Those related to the element of Water would tend to cause a delayed reaction just as water tends to linger on until it evaporates. While those related to the element of Wind would only cause death when the arrow or spear was removed. In all of the above cases, the surgeon needed to know these points and their effects in order to be effective. Also, surgery on marmas could be a risky enterprise if the surgeon was not aware of them.

A surgical operation where the incision leaves a scar across various channels can interfere with the channels' energy conduction and promote ill health in the local area as well as in remote areas. For instance, a horizontal hysterectomy scar below the navel can interfere with the kidney, stomach, conception and other channels' pranic flow.

It is also interesting to note that today, it has been found that a vaccination in the arm at a marma point can produce a delayed effect of chronic proportions for the young patient. Whereas if injected not at the particular point, the effect would be lessened.

As a side-line, the late martial arts expert Bruce Lee is believed by many to have received a blow to one of the delayed marmas which subsequently caused him to die from a brain hemorrhage. Since Bruce was superbly fit, it is possible that this effect actually caused his unusual type of death for such a healthy man.

Professor Dr. P.H.Kulkarni states:

> *"the extremity marmas [reflex points] are not very dangerous and hence none of them are described under Sadyah Pranhar category."* [13]

This tends to point to additional marmas which by their own inherent not-so-dangerous nature are unclassified by Charaka. These include the ones found near the fingers and toes and are extremely important for Ayurvedic Acupuncture, even if not so important for surgery. These will be explained in the text to follow.

CHANNELS *(Nadis)*

Thus far, Ayurveda contains not only a system of needling (in common with surgery) but also one that incorporates reflex or vital points (marmas). A true system of acupuncture must also have a system of channels (which the Chinese call meridians) located underneath the skin, which connect with the points or marmas and also with major human organs (e.g. the heart and its channel). Charaka once again explains:

> *"Of all these, some varieties of (important) channels will be described here with reference to their controlling organs and also the symptoms manifested by their vitiation. This description will be sufficient for an ignorant man to understand the characteristic features of these channels, while for a wise man,* **this description will provide enough material enabling him to understand the characteristic features of other channels which are not described here.** *As long as these channels perform their normal functions, the body is free from disease."* [14]

Of course, some of these channels are physical like the arteries which carry blood and others are invisible like the energy channels. Charaka further explains this:

> *"Srotas ([gross] channel), vein (sira), artery (dhamani), Lymphatic channel (rasayani) and energy channel or duct (nadi) . . . these are the names attributed to visible and invisible spaces inside the tissue elements of the body."* [15]

The channels which relate to physical substances like blood are normally called Srotas, whereas the ones carrying the life-energy are called Nadis.

Yoga expert and teacher B.K.S. Iyengar explains:

> *"It is said in the* Varahopanishad *(V,54/5) that the Nadis (channels) penetrate the body from the soles of the feet to the crown of the head. In them is Prana, the breath of life."* [16]

MAJOR ORGANS *(Kosthangas)*
Charaka also outlined the major human organs as detailed in the Sharirasthana chapter of the Charaka Samhitta. He states:

> *"Kosthangas (organs in the thorax and abdomen) are:*

Heart (hrdaya)	Kidney (vrkkau)
Lung (kloman)	Urinary Bladder (hasti)
Liver (yakrt)	Gall bladder
Large Intestine (sthulantra)	Spleen (pliha)
Stomach (amashaya)	Small intestine (ksudantra)." [17]

These ten organs, plus the Pericardium and Tridosha (both considered organs in Ayurveda) form the twelve major organs which have Acupuncture channels in the body (e.g. the Heart, Liver, Kidney Channels etc.).

LIFE-FORCE *(Prana)*
No acupuncture system, even though containing the above mentioned requirements, can truly be acupuncture without consideration

of the most important ingredient. That ingredient is the bio-energy which the Chinese call Chi, the Koreans and Japanese call Ki and the Indians call Prana.

Ayurvedic expert Dr. Bhagwan Dash explains:

> Prana is the "Life-force, elan vital."[18]

B.K.S. Iyengar says that:

> "Prana is the energy permeating the universe at all levels. It is physical, mental, intellectual, sexual, spiritual and cosmic energy. It is the prime mover of all activity. It is energy which creates, protects and destroys. Vigor, power, vitality, life are all forms of Prana."[19]

By inhaling or via food/drinks, Prana is carried into the body via oxygen molecules. Prana then circulates via innumerable channels, including the classical Ida and Pingala channels of Yoga, and concentrates around the Chakras or bio-energy flywheels of the body. Prana also circulates through the channels which directly connect with the human organs described by Charaka. It is because of the pranic flow of energy that tissues, organs and structures remain alive, since without it they would perish (as in the case of gangrene—which lacks Prana).

ACUPUNCTURE BASIS

It is unfortunate that many traditional Ayurvedic practices have remained secretive and have all but disappeared from popular usage. This has been attributed in most cases to the various invasions of India and also due to natural calamities.

As an example, there is a system of martial arts in India called Marma Adi (a part of Kalari) which is the secretive and complex art of striking vital pressure points for self-defense purposes. It is still kept quite secret, even in India, and very little information is available today to the West. It is estimated that about one million Indians practice this form of martial art but since India is such a large continent and it has an extremely dense population (900 million plus), this represents an extremely small percentage of the population who know about this art. It is difficult to find a true master or Gurukal from among such a sea of people.

Marma Adi's secrets were recorded in 72 shastras or ancient books which were written on palm leaf manuscripts and carefully handed down many generations from a master to his most trusted pupil. This knowledge was reputedly given by Agastya to eighteen of his most trusted students who each wrote four of the 72 works. To date, only 40 of these valuable manuscripts remain and are in a process of modern translation by martial arts scholar Moses Thilak of Madras. These books, on loan to Moses by very traditional practitioners of not only self-defense but also Ayurvedic medicine, contain explicit information about vital points, methods of healing and striking these vital points, and other secretive information.

Likewise, many diagnostic and therapeutic procedures and art forms have almost all but disappeared from popular use in India. Ayurvedic acupuncture and moxibustion appear to be two of these systems, although once again they are gaining popularity, even if only very gradually.

Dr. Chandrashekkar G. Thakkur (world famous authority on Ayurvedic medicine) states that:

> *"in India, acupuncture was in use several millennia before Christ and is still flourishing today."* [20]

The Ayurvedic acupuncture form is termed *BhedanKarma* (piercing through therapy) and is a part of the Suchi Veda or the science of needling, according to Ayurvedic principles.

> *"Needling ear points was recorded in an ancient Indian text, the Suchi Veda (science of needling) about 3000 years ago."* [21]

Although Ayurvedic Acupuncture is today not as popularly practiced as its Chinese counterpart, it is a science worth studying. It forms an intricate part of Ayurvedic knowledge, fulfilling Ayurveda as a complete system. Ayurvedic acupuncture should perhaps be

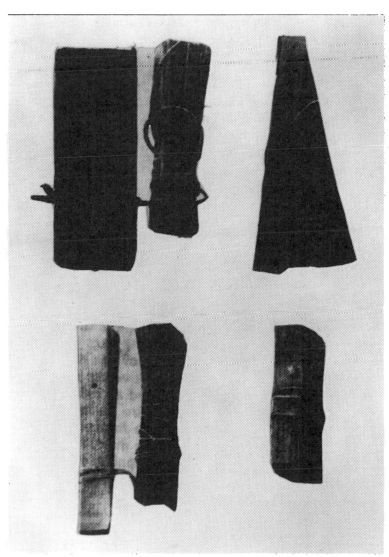

Kalari Shastras

taught as a post-graduate Ayurvedic course in the West.
Drs. Vasant Lad and David Frawley explain it well when they state:

> "Ayurveda means 'The Science of Life'. It is a science of living that encom-
> passes the whole of life, and which relates the life of the individual to that
> of the universe. As such it is open to and includes all life, and all methods
> that bring us into greater harmony with life. It is one with all life, a knowledge
> that belongs to all living beings—not a system imposed upon them, but a
> resource to be drawn upon freely and to be adapted to the unique needs of
> the individual in his or her particular environment."[22]

Notes:

1. *Acupuncture*, p. 1.
2. *Science and Secrets of Early Medicine*, p. 206.
3. *Acupuncture Marma and Other Asian Therapeutic Techniques*, pp. iv-v.
4. *Charaka Samhitta*, p. 412.
5. *A Modern Guide to Ear Acupuncture*, p. 187.
6. *Charaka*, p. xxi
7. *Links Between Ayureveda and Acupuncture*, p. 1.
8. *Donden*, p. 7.
9. *Ibid.*, p. 25.
10. *Charaka*, p. 457.
11. *Acupuncture Marma and Other Asian Therapeutic Techniques*, p. 37.
12. *Acupuncture Marma*, pp. 4-5.
13. *Links Between Acupuncture and Ayurveda*, p. 7.
14. *Charaka Samhitta*, p. 173
15. *Ibid.*, p. 177.
16. *Light on Pranayama*, p. 33.
17. *Charaka Samhitta*, Vol. II VII, pp. 454-455.
18. *Ayurveda for Mother and Child*, p. 156.
19. *Light on Pranayama*, p. 12.
20. *Modern Guide to Ear Acupuncture*, p. 4.
21. Callinan, *Australian Wellbeing*, Vol. 31.
22. *Yoga of Herbs*, p. 2.

CHAPTER II
PART I

THE FIVE ELEMENTS

Ayurveda recognizes five physical elements which are part of everything. Each object is different because it possesses the elements in varying ratios in comparison to other objects. These Five Elements called Pancha Mahabhutas (the Five Great Elements) are the underlying elements of all structures. Some of these are very physical like water and earth, others are less physical like fire, wind or ether.

A rock, for instance, has a majority of earth, but it also must have a certain amount of water to provide cohesion between the earth particles. It also has fire (probably received from the Sun) which baked it into shape. Without fire, the rock would be totally freezing in temperature. Likewise, since science believes that nothing is solid but that atomically every solid substance has gaps between the particles, there must similarly be air within the particles of the rock. So a rock, like other objects, contains these five elements.

A living being, that is an animal or human, has an additional element to the five already mentioned. That is the element of Prana or bio-energy. It is this energy which provides life and animation to the object. A dead animal has therefore lost this essential life-energy, although the other five still remain in one form or another.

Essentially, Prana is the first universal energetic element which provides and supports life. Just as electricity (energy) requires a conduit by which to work (cable), so does Prana (bio-energy) require a physical conduit (body) which is made up of the Five Elements.

Einstein explained by his famous equation of $E=MC^2$ that energy and matter are interchangeable, matter being a more compressed form of energy. Matter, therefore, vibrates at a different frequency to energy; but both have similar origins.

Ayurveda also explains that everything started in energy (Prana) and that through a process of creation, the other five (matter) elements were created. So that energy and matter are simply different frequencies of the same primordial energy (Prana).

Ayurveda maintains that the soul contains Prana and has traditionally interchanged these two terms.

Although this concept made no difference when religion and medicine were intertwined in the ancient days, there is a reason today for separating the connotation of the soul (which can be construed as a religious concept) from the idea of Prana (bio-energy). These two appear to have a common denominator but they are both different aspects of human life.

Dr. Bhagwan Dash explains that Prana is life-energy, and it must be present at the point of birth. Yet he also states that according to Vagbhata, the soul enters the human fetus during the fifth month of pregnancy. [1] That is five months after the fetus has received Prana. So it is logical that Prana and the Soul are two different, although related entities. Charaka, the ancient Ayurvedic master explained the soul (consciousness) as Prana and vice-versa. This is what he says about the subject:

> *"The Soul [including Prana], first of all unites with Ether (akasha) before uniting with the other elements [bhutas] . . . whose attributes are more and more manifested successively."* [2]

Creation Of The Cosmos

According to Ayurveda, the combination of Prana (energy) and Ether (matter called Akasha) created movement, for energy needs matter for physical action to occur. Electricity needs a cable to be conducted to the light globe.

Ayurveda calls this action or movement Wind (Vayu), since wind has the characteristic of movement. Through Wind (or movement) against matter, friction arose which caused Fire (heat). This Fire heated some of the matter particles to the point of melting (liquefaction) and thereby caused Water to flow. The combination of water with matter formed a solidification later resulting in Earth. The cosmos was then fully formed.

Human Creation

Besides the creation of the cosmos by Prana via the Five Elements (Pancha Mahabhutas), the process of creation appears each time a baby is born. This is termed the Wheel of Creation, where each element successively allows the creation of a living being. Charaka once again describes this cycle or wheel when he states:

> *"The embryo is formed by the five mahabhutas [elements] viz. Ether, Wind, Fire, Water and Earth and it serves as a receptacle of consciousness. In fact, the Soul (i.e. conscious element [inc. Prana]) constitutes the sixth element responsible for the formation of the embryo."*[3]

Consequently, Charaka explains that there are six elements, Ether, Wind, Fire, Water, Earth and Prana. The five physical elements then serve as a receptacle for Prana or life energy and subsequently for the conscious element or soul (the latter being received at the fifth month of pregnancy).

Energy (Prana) is bestowed the function of driving force or positive action in the body. Prana like electricity is the one that flows through the body and is regarded as the positive side of the equation.

Ether, on the other hand, is the first physical element which interfaces directly with Prana (according to Charaka) and is therefore considered the negative force or part of the equation. Just like a battery needs a positive and a negative terminal to be functional, so too Prana(+) and Ether (Akasha)(-) are needed. Ayurveda believes that a human male has more positive energy than a female who then has more negative energy than the male. Consequently, more males suffer heart attacks (related to positive/heat energy) than the females, who suffer more nervous disorders (negative energy). The male is considered more Pitta (positive energy) while the female is considered more Kapha/Vata (negative energy).

In the process of human reproduction Prana {+} (male) joins with Ether {-} (female) by coitus. Through the movement of coitus which is related to Wind, friction arises which causes heat/perspiration etc. which is related to Fire. When orgasm occurs semen is ejaculated

(Water). This semen then joins the ovum to form a zygote—(conception) which is the process of solidification (Earth).

ELEMENT	OCCURRENCE
Prana (+)	Male
Ether (-)	Akasha Female
Wind	Coition (movement)
Fire	Orgasm (friction)
Water	Ejaculation (semen) liquefaction
Earth	Conception (zygote) solidification

The elements' appearance is therefore from the least physical (more subtle) Ether, to the most physical, that is Earth.

The Wheel of Creation represents not only the formation of the cosmos and the process of childbirth, but also the creation of the Five Elements themselves. Prana or elementary life energy therefore underwrites all of life's processes.

Creation of the Three Humors
Each element thus appeared in a certain sequence, referred to as the Wheel of Creation. This also led to the creation of other physical forces and organs in the human body. As Dr. David Frawley explains:

> "The physical body is a manifestation of our life-force [Prana]; imbalances in the life-force produce disease. The biological humors [Vata, Pitta, Kapha] are merely three different statuses or orientations of the life-force."[4]

VATA
The combination of Ether and Wind (via Prana) caused a type of energy or humor to be created. This is termed Vata which is related to the word Vayu or Wind. Vata is the most subtle humor and is normally involved in most physical maladies, because being closer to the source of energy, it is easier to unbalance. Vata is considered the catabolic humor.

Professor Dr. P.H. Kulkarni explains that "Abnormal Vata humor has been described as the main cause for all diseases in the body." [5]

Vata has certain physical characteristics, so that when it becomes unbalanced, these show up as dryness (of skin and other parts) and anxiety, nervous reactions, especially aggravated by cold wind. Most Vata disorders first appear below the navel as this is the site of this humor (see Fig. 1). Vata, like the other two humors, is inherited so that a person may be prone to certain Vata disorders unless preventive measures are taken. By this, Vata is also a constitution, with a proneness to certain diseases.

PITTA

The next two elements to appear—Fire and Water—equate with the formation of Pitta, the Ayurvedic heat humor. Pitta is really Prana plus Fire and Water since the bio-energy is required at all stages of life. Pitta is the second most subtle humor and is involved in metabolism or formation since fire tends to shape things. Pitta is the metabolic humor and is related to the hormonal system.

Pitta is the middle humor and as such involves heat which is essentially obtained from combustion during digestion. Pitta imbalances can be recognized due to redness, heat, rashes and inflammation of various parts of the body.

KAPHA

The last two elements are Water and Earth. These two (with Prana) form the Kapha humor which deals with growth (anabolism) in the body. The combination of water and earth results in mud and so when Kapha is aggravated, loose joints can occur and weight can easily be gained (fat is much like water and earth).

Kapha is translated by Charaka as "phlegm" (water and earth) so that its imbalance may result in heaviness, congestion and lack of flow. Kapha represents growth, sometimes through muscles and sometimes through excess fat. Obesity is therefore a Kapha disorder. Excessive muscle size (e.g. induced by anabolic steroids) is also a Kapha disorder

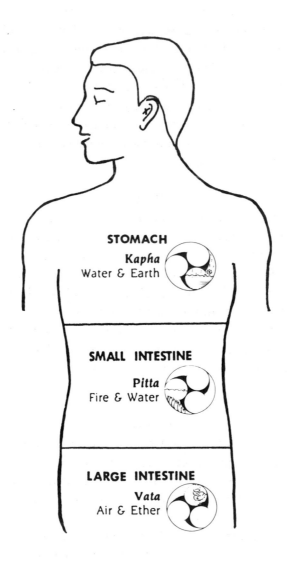

Fig. 1 Sites of the three humors *(Tridoshas)*

while abundance of hair is usually a Kapha feature. Kapha is normally regarded as centering above the breathing diaphragm or area of the chest. As such, Ayurveda regards this area as the Kapha area and many Kapha disorders originate there. Phlegm is a human secretion which is connected with Kapha.

Ayurveda classifies the organs and tissues according to the Five Elements. For instance, due to the fact that bile, blood and urine contain much water, these three have a strong obvious relationship with the Water element (jala). Some organs, like the small intestine, the stomach, urinary and gall bladders and the large intestine are considered hollow organs ("containing space"). They are therefore classified as ethereal organs since Ether is also translated as "space". Bones and muscles are considered Earth tissues, since they are solid structures, a feature of the Earth element. This is the simple basis by which many ideas are explained.

Besides this idea, Ayurveda also explains that each major organ (and tissue) of the body is also related to one of the Five Elements in a sophisticated and logical form, since without the elements, these organs etc. would not exist. The relationship between them is not only of a simple, physically obvious nature but it also encompasses connection via the subtle body, via the Nadis or bio-energy channels.

FIRE *(Teja)*
The element of Fire provides shaping of a substance but it has no physical form. When the fuel is removed, fire tends to go out. Furthermore you are neither able to grasp fire nor retain it without fuel.

Ayurveda classifies the small intestine (S.I.) as a hollow organ and the primary site of aggravation when Pitta (the heat humor) becomes unbalanced. It is in this organ that Pitta problems usually originate and then migrate to other parts of the body to where they reflect Pitta's characteristic morbidity.

The Pitta humor is considered in Ayurveda as having Fire and Water in greater proportion than the other three elements. The main characteristic of this humor is not fluid retention caused by a buildup of water but rather heat. Ayurveda calls this heat Fire. The main protagonist in Pitta is therefore fire, which represents all things of a hot nature, whether they be hyperacidity, red rashes or inflammation. The small intestine, the site of Pitta, has therefore a subtle connection with the Fire element, through its Pitta characteristics. Ayurveda also relates that *Agni*, the digestive heat, is found in the small intestine.

Ayurveda considers the blood to be primarily a Pitta tissue. Blood and blood vessels have a strong relationship with Pitta and therefore with Fire, Pitta's main and primary element. Pitta or heat is carried by the blood to all parts of the body. There is one organ whose main function is to pump blood around the body; it controls the flow of blood. Its interaction with blood and Pitta is undeniable. This organ is the heart.

Dr. David Frawley explains that heart attacks relate to Pitta which obviously relate to the Fire element:

> *"In the Ayurvedic association of Pitta (fire) with the blood, heart disease, particularly heart attacks and strokes, is commonly a Pitta disorder. The [person] who suddenly dies of a heart attack, is typically a Pitta person who denies his true heart."* [6]

It is obvious then, that the small intestine and the heart are two Pitta-related organs. Consequently, both of these organs have a fundamental connection with the Fire element. In Ayurvedic acupuncture, where this knowledge is absolutely necessary, the interconnection between the heart and small intestine as Fire and Pitta organs, is important.

EARTH *(Prithvi)*

The Earth element is the solid state of matter and the basis on which most physical things are built. It provides stability and allows growth. The Earth element is a major component of the Kapha humor.

The Kapha humor is aggravated in the stomach according to classical Ayurveda. When Kapha is aggravated, the stomach is the site of accumulation, and later migrating to other sites of the body where it reproduces its characteristic symptoms of morbidity. For example, phlegm (earth + water) first accumulates in the stomach and later attacks the lungs and respiratory system.

Kapha's main attributes or characteristics are heaviness, congestion and lack of flow. Picture a pipe carrying water to a distant location. Then gradually add more and more Earth or (sand) to the water. The flow will gradually be restricted and congestion will set in. The total weight of the pipe and contents will increase dramatically due to the excess earth (heaviness). There will also be a lack of flow of water through the pipe. These characteristics were not created by water, which would allow free flow but rather by earth. Earth causes congestion when there is more of it than water. This results in rigidity and lack of flow.

So too, Kapha's main protagonist is Earth. Kapha is made up of Earth (and water) so that if Kapha originates in the stomach, then the stomach must also be related to the Earth element (which is a part of phlegm, anyway).

The spleen is regarded in many cases as a Pitta organ because it retains blood so as to supply it in an emergency (e.g. hemorrhaging). The truth is that the spleen is an Earth element related organ since it controls muscle growth and in conjunction with the pancreas (which controls fat growth), both relate to Kapha. It is well known that the pancreas affects sugar levels in the body. An imbalance in any of these three organs results in a Kapha disorder, either excess muscle, excess fat or excess phlegm. This idea is validated by Ayurvedic pulse diagnosis where the common connection of Earth places the spleen and stomach at the same radial artery position. The stomach is detected by superficial pressure of the middle finger, while the spleen and pancreas are detected by deep pressure at the same position. Dr. Lad fully elucidates this concept in his book *Ayurveda, The Science of Self-Healing*. Also, the spleen is anatomically positioned on the left side of the body, the negative Kapha side according to Ayurveda, while the liver is placed on the right, positive Pitta side of the body.

WIND *(Vayu)*

The Ayurvedic concept of Wind is that of air which creates movement. It is not one of stagnant air. Wind is the gaseous state of matter. Air consists of Prana, mostly carried by oxygen molecules and is the energy which keeps everything alive. Like every other object in the universe, it also consists of Ether which is the physical space or matrix in which to house Prana. Ether's primary qualities are somewhat akin to space and matter.

We prefer to call this element Wind instead of air because the former has an attribute of movement; whereas the latter can be stagnant. These two terms are often interchangeable in Ayurveda.

Air is breathed in through the lungs, so this organ must be related to the Wind element. Prana also enters the lungs via the air which is inhaled and is then distributed throughout the body. One of the meanings of Prana (from *"an"*, meaning to breathe) is "breathing". Prana, carried by air outside and within the body is referred to as Vayu, which means Wind.

Another way that Prana enters the body is via fresh foods like fruits and vegetables since plants like humans also utilize Prana. The large intestine is the site where Ayurveda believes that Prana from foods is extracted and absorbed into the body. The large intestine is also the site where wind (abdominal gas) is generated and from where it is expelled.

Ayurvedic physician Dr. Robert Svoboda says that:

> *"We obtain Prana from our atmosphere and from our food. Prana is the life force; oxygen is one of its carrier substances. Breathing [correctly] recharges Prana immediately. Prana is absorbed from the colon [large intestine]."*[7]

So consequently the lung and large intestine energetically connected together are related to Wind (and Prana) and:

> *"Pathologies in the lungs and large intestine are often related, balancing one of these organs can benefit the other."*[8]

Wind is the element of movement and directly affects and is

affected by the lung and large intestine. As a consequence, it affects the nerves as well, so that a person with excess Wind element in their system can be easily agitated by a cold wind.

WATER *(Jala)*

The Water element is extremely important, for it allows correct flow within the body. The human body is composed of approximately 70% water. Water provides cohesion for the other elements and by itself is not stable.

Water is also a medium for Prana. Rain water collects Prana as it falls from the clouds. Dr. Svoboda says that "water also carries Prana." [8] The flow of Prana through the body resembles the flow of water, which is the element of flux.

Although some of the water is excreted by the body via the skin during perspiration, most of it is removed from the body by the kidneys (and urinary bladder). The kidney and the Water element must therefore be interrelated. Water forms an important part of Kapha along with Earth so that when water is retained in the body (fluid retention), another type of Kapha imbalance is formed. It may cause looseness of body joints, perhaps in the knees and ankles, and generally will result in congestion.

Of course, the function of the kidneys is not only to retain water (fluid) in the body when desired or when there is an imbalance, but also it has a very strong function of removing water (via urine) when there is excess. For instance, in summer, when heat is great, water is retained naturally in the body to reduce the body temperature to its balance position (37° C). In winter, when there is excess cold, the body (via the kidneys) will eliminate excess water in order to increase the body temperature to its balance position.

So the kidneys have a dual role, one of retaining water in the body which equates to Kapha and one of eliminating water where necessary, which equates to Vata (dryness). Of course an imbalance in the kidneys can result in either Vata or Kapha symptoms, depending on whether there is an excess or deficiency of water in the body.

The urinary bladder is the hollow sack which receives urine from the kidneys after this organ has filtered impurities and water from the blood. The urinary bladder and the kidney not only have a strong interrelationship due to the anatomical connection between them (by the pipes known as the ureters), but also due to their energy connection via the Water element.

ETHER *(Akasha)*

Ether is the most subtle of the Five Elements. Ether (Akasha) not only means space and matter but it is also translated as:

> "**ETHER** (Greek = *aither* = to burn) an invisible substance postulated as pervading space and transmitting radiant energy." [9]

Ether is the most difficult element to come to terms with in Ayurveda. Since one of the meanings of Akasha (Ether) is "sound", then it is normal for Ayurveda to relate it to Vata (the Wind humor) which also relates to sound. In order to prevent any confusion from arising, it should be made clear that Ether does indeed directly relate to Vata. It is one of the two main elements of Vata, along with Wind.

Dr. R. Svoboda describes Ether as: *"the field from which everything is manifested and into which everything returns; the space in which events occur."* [10]

Dr. Bhagwan Dash and Professor Manfred Junius describe Akasha (Ether) from the Sanskrit *"root: Kash [5] 'to radiate', that which does not provide resistance."* [11]

The English word *Ether* is used as a direct translation from the Sanskrit because of the true reflection of its Ayurvedic meaning. It exhibits the same qualities which the ancients regarded as Akasha. On the one hand, Ether has cold and dry attributes, on a par with the Vata humor. On the other hand, it also has a potential energy which, when released, can "radiate" and become totally different from its previous qualities.

In chemistry, ether is related to alcohol, an organic compound obtained from ethanol and sulfuric acid and which was used as an anesthetic. Ethanol is a colorless, flammable alcohol and as such directly relates to Ether. Alcohol's qualities, on its own (when in a jar), are cooling and drying. By placing a small quantity of alcohol on the skin, these two qualities become fully evident. A dry, cool feeling is noticed around the area.

Liver Fire (BhutaAgni)

Alcohol's other quality is one of heating, since when it is lit by a match, it will ignite brightly and release heat. In the human body, Ether is affected by 37° C. of heat which is the body's normal internal temperature. This temperature would be considered high if outside of the body (environmental weather). This heat (which is found firstly in the small intestine and called Agni) tends to heat up the Ether. Later, when the Ether element (e.g. from food) is digested and transformed in the liver into body-type Ether, the BhutaAgnis (the Five Element Fires) ignite this Ether to produce heat in the liver. Since Ether, like timber, is the only one of the Five Elements which has the potential to ignite, it loses its cold attributes when digested in the body.

Ether therefore, relates to Pitta, the heat humor, while the liver (and its related gallbladder) is a Pitta organ.

The main effect of alcohol (and Ether) is one of drying as when alcohol is consumed by a person. The after-effect of alcohol tends to be extreme thirst "in the morning". A secondary but most important after-effect is the destruction of the liver by prolonged use of alcohol, causing cirrhosis or scarring of the liver. Consequently, alcohol (and ether) causes dryness (like Vata) but also causes heat (like Pitta).

Ether has a cool and dry effect as part of Vata, due to its connection with "space and matter", but it also has a heating quality which is released in the body by the liver, and is related to Pitta. Bile, a product released by the liver and stored in the gall bladder is, in fact, one of the translations of Pitta. Dr. Vasant Lad confirms that the liver and Pitta are related on page 42, in *Ayurveda—The Science Of Self-Healing.*

The Five Elements described herein are the underlying basis of all things and along with Prana, explain Ayurvedic acupuncture. Each humor, tissue, organ, etc. therefore has a relationship with the Five Elements and Prana.

Interestingly, although the Five Elements have been recorded in Ayurveda since time immemorial, and are extremely important for a true understanding of Ayurvedic acupuncture, they seem to have been missing from Chinese medicine until late in the third century B.C.

Experts in Oriental medicine and its history, Professor P. Huard, professor at the Medical Faculty, Paris and Dr. Ming Wong, of the Medical Faculty at Rennes, are both members of the International Academy of the History of Medicine and are leading authorities on Eastern Medicine.

Professor Huard and Dr. Wong in their book *Chinese Medicine* state:

> *"From this period onwards [circa 300 B.C.] China borrowed from India and Iran. Thus Tsou Yen (c. 305-240 B.C.) introduced to the Far East the idea of the five elements, their mutual genesis and destruction, after which the Chinese medical system was built upon the doctrine of the elements."* [12]

Also they mention that prior to this period, Chinese medicine functioned mainly by the basic concept of the two opposites and not by the Five Elements. This duality concept, although called Yin and Yang in Chinese, was also shared by most other cultures including India and Egypt, since most knew the natural concepts of Sun-Moon, light-dark, male-female, left-right, etc. In India, this interrelationship between all things is termed *Dvandva* (or duality) and has formed part of Ayurveda.

> *"The Chinese hypotheses [prior to Tsou Yen], referred only to the two principles and eight triagrams to account for the perpetual transformation of things.*
> *Tsou Yen tried to amalgamate ideas of Chinese origin with new Western notions which he probably received from Indian travellers, that of the five elements and their gyration and of the reciprocal destruction and genesis of*

the five natural agents." [13]

According to Chinese experts, the earliest record of medicine in China in which acupuncture and the Five Elements are mentioned is from about the period of Tsou Yen. This was after a huge influx into the country of Indian ideas and philosophies brought about by a vital movement of a new Indian religious philosophy—Buddhism (c. 563 B.C.). This tends to reaffirm the above facts.

> *"The earliest extant medical classic in China,* Huangdi Neijing *(Canon of Medicine) was compiled between 500-300 B.C. The book, which consists of two parts, describes the basic theories of traditional Chinese medicine, such as yin-yang, the five elements, solid-hollow organs, channels . . . "* [14]

For the last two thousand years or so, the Chinese have used the concepts of Ayurveda, integrating them into their system of medicine. Today, it has become an homogenous whole. Their efforts in popularizing these concepts throughout the ancient Orient are renowned, in much the same way they did with Buddhism (Zen). Countries like Japan, Korea, Vietnam and most others in the Orient have greatly benefitted from the desire to spread these concepts beyond their own borders. In more recent times, they have been very influential in spreading the doctrine of oriental medicine, specifically acupuncture, to most corners of the West and have helped the cause of natural therapies and their general acceptance throughout the world. The Chinese people are therefore to be wholeheartedly congratulated.

Ayurvedic acupuncture can only be truly explained by a knowledge of the Five Elements, since they also demonstrate the connection between each organ, e.g. Wind-Lung/Large Intestine. The elements also explain why the organ channels are located where they are along the body. For instance, the Wind element explains that the Lung channel and the Large Intestine channel (nadis) must be located along the same limb, since they are interrelated. Also, the elements explain the radial pulses as found in Ayurveda and its related Tibetan medical system. It is by Wind that the lung and large intestine can be detected

on the same radial position by the same index finger. Since the
elements are the basis of all things, then it is logical that their actions
and interactions (Wheels) explain Ayurveda and acupuncture.

PART II

ELEMENT SYNDROMES

Imbalances of the Five Elements in the human body can produce
various signs and symptoms according to the element's characteristics
or attributes called *Guna-Dvandva* (duality of attributes). Guna-
Dvandva is described by Charaka, the ancient Ayurvedic physician
in his text (XXVI [10]), which outlines ten pairs of said attributes by
which to diagnose and treat patients.

For instance, dryness of the skin can be treated by its opposite
quality—oiliness. A hot type of syndrome (Pitta) can be reduced by
its opposite—coldness (Kapha).

The Element syndromes are symptoms which explain medical imbalance or disease. It often occurs prior to a full-blown disease and
therefore can form a very important part of prevention.

Fire

An imbalance in Fire generally means too much Fire (or heat) exists
in the body. When this occurs, symptoms like hyperacidity, high blood
heat, red skin rashes, inflamed tissues or joints, excessive perspiration,
fever, irritability, yellow urine and excessive thirst may be evident. This
condition has similar characteristics to a Pitta disorder, since Pitta
contains heat.

A deficiency of Fire in the body would allow coldness to set in and
demonstrate paleness of skin etc. The digestive fire (Agni) would
similarly suffer, thus causing malabsorption of nutrients and accumulation of toxins (Ama) in the body.

Earth

An excess of Earth would mean coldness, congestion, rigidity, heaviness and lack of flow. Symptoms include lethargy, loss of appetite, heaviness in limbs, lack of circulation and rigidity of joints, pallor, nausea and excess sleeping. This is similar to a high Kapha (Earth) imbalance.

A deficiency of Earth on the other hand would cause muscles to lose their tone, bones to lose calcium and become weak. Generally the body structure would lose its strength. This would equate with a high Vata condition

Wind

An imbalance in the function of Wind would allow excess dryness of the skin, other tissues and joints, coldness and high sensitivity to wind, lack of circulation due to drying of moisture in the blood, abdominal distention, constipation, fear, fatigue, insomnia, spasms, borborygmus, pain and stiffness of joints, lower back pains and dry coughs.

A deficiency of Wind would result in loss of Prana, congestion and waterlogging. The symptoms would be similar to a high Kapha imbalance.

Water

An excess of Water would allow water-logging of the tissues and joints. There would also be an increase in heaviness of the limbs, bloating, increased salivation, phlegm, productive coughs, glands which are swollen, the swelling of joints and low fevers.

Ether

The Ether described in these syndromes relates to Pitta, where an excess would affect the liver and produce bitter taste in the mouth. Also anger, conjunctivitis, bilious vomiting and diarrhea with burning feelings would reflect an excess of Ether..

A deficiency of Ether or energy in the liver can cause a loss of bile and digestive disorders.

Where Ether is described as cold and dry, the symptoms would be like Vata disorders.

Notes:

1. *Ayurveda For Mother And Child*, p. 9.
2. *Charaka Samhitta*, p. 390.
3. *Ibid.*, p. 388.
4. *Ayurvedic Healing*, p. 108.
5. Kulkarni, p. 9.
6. *Ayurvedic Healing*, p. 170.
7. Svoboda, p. 124.
8. *Prakruti— Your Ayurvedic Constitution*, p. 124.
9. *Collins Australian Dictionary*.
10. *Prakruti— Your Ayurvedic Constitution*, p. 17.
11. *A Handbook of Ayurveda*, p. 14.
12. *Chinese Medicine*, p. 12.
13. *Ibid.*, pp. 88-89,
14. *Essentials of Chinese Acupuncture*, pp. 5-6.

CHAPTER III

THE BIO-ENERGY CHANNELS

CHANNELS *(Nadis)*

The type of channel which Ayurveda calls *Srota* differs from a Nadi in that the former is a pipe or channel which carries mostly physical fluids like blood, plasma, lymph, etc. (e.g. arteries, lymph ducts), while the latter is a conduit or duct for the flow of subtle Prana or life energy. The Nadis (or subtle channels), having a direct relationship with Prana, modify the flow of fluids through the gross channels or Srotas in a parallel fashion. When the Nadis' energy flow is impaired, the Srota's flow will similarly be affected. The *Charaka Samhitta* refers to the Srotas as the "channels of circulation", also denoting them as gross channels in contrast with the Nadis.

Professor Dr. P.H. Kulkarni, Poona University Research Guide explains:

> *"The concept of [Pranic] meridians runs parallel with the Yogic Nadis [channels] rather than the Srotas. Some of the Chakras described in Yoga may also have interesting correlations with acupuncture meridians and points."*[1]

Dr. Kim Bong Han, from the North Korean University of Pyongang, found after extensive research that the energy channels are composed of a special type of histological tissue as yet not noticed by Science but which provides a pathway for life-energy. Dr. Kim adds that the channels have a thin membranous wall and contain transparent and colorless liquid.

Restriction of Prana through the nadis will result in the impedance in the flow of fluids through the srota channels. So that the underlying fault in most diseases is a malfunction in the flow of Prana. Prana, life-energy, is a component of the Vata humor and it is indeed Prana working through the body (akasha) which is termed Vata. It is through the medium of the external Vayu or Wind that Prana enters the body to become Vata humor.

"*Abnormal Vata humor has been described as the main cause for all diseases in the body. The therapeutic efficacy of Acupuncture will thus be required to be considered in the light of abnormal Vata humor in various diseases.*"[2]

Pitta and Kapha are totally lame humors (or forces) without the assistance of Vata (containing Prana) in the body. Vata equates with movement and it forces the other two opposites—Pitta (heat) and Kapha (cold)—to move and perform, just like the wind forces fire and water (sea and rain) to move about. The Nadi and Prana concepts are also still retained in the ancient science of Yoga and forms a very important and integral part of its philosophy. Dr. Vasant Lad says:

"*The beats of the pulse reveal something about the important meridians (nadi channels) that are connecting Pranic currents of energy in the body, passing through the vital organs such as the liver, kidney etc.*"[3]

We have previously confirmed that each major organ in the body is related to another one via one of the Five Elements. The organs (heart and small intestine) are interrelated through the connection of the Fire element and the nadis or channels which emanate from both organs. Prana leaves the heart (a solid organ) and travels through the Heart channel to connect with the Small Intestine channel. The Small Intestine channel then appropriately connects with another channel to continue the free flow of Prana throughout the body. These channels which relate to each of the twelve organs, form a loop (or daisy chain) so that Prana continues its circulation through the body, completing its journey every twenty-four hours.

The channels (nadis) are located in the body according to a logical scheme, a natural law at work (see Fig. 2). These channels are positioned in the body according to two criteria.

1. The organ's physical position in the human trunk if the organ is a solid (major) type.

2. The location is according to the organ's element connection if the organ is a hollow type.

There are six organs which Ayurveda regards as solid, totally essential and cannot be removed from the body (today they may be

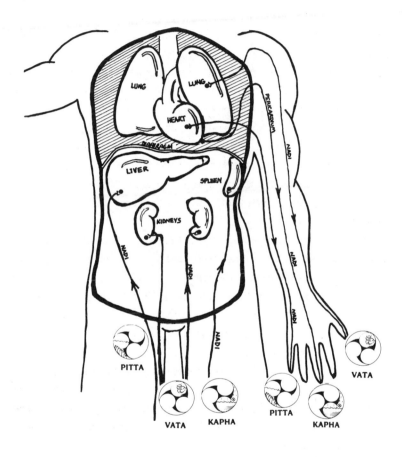

Fig. 2 The organ channels and their relationship with Tridoshas

transplanted). They are the heart, lung, kidney, liver, spleen (also pancreas) and pericardium (more of this organ later). The physical anatomical positions of these organs correlate to the physical position of their channels in the body. Where one of these six organs is located above the breathing diaphragm, protected by the rib cage (thorax), its channel is similarly located above the diaphragm. In this case, the channels then meander from their related organs along the arm (upper limb) to reach the fingers.

Where the organ is anatomically positioned below the diaphragm, its related channel is located along the lower limb—the leg.

Of the six solid organs described above, three are located in the thoracic area (above the diaphragm). These are the heart, lung and pericardium (which surrounds the heart). Their channels are then located along the arm.

The three remaining solid organs below the thorax are the liver, kidney and spleen. Their channels must logically be found meandering along the lower limb—the leg.

The six hollow organs have their channels according to the organ's element connection. The small intestine, which relates to the element of Fire, has its channel adjacent to the Heart channel, along the arm. The heart is another Fire organ.

The large intestine is related to the element of Wind and consequently its channel is located adjacent to the other Wind organ—the lung, which has its channel along the arm. This scheme applies to the other organs which similarly are related to the elements. Their description follows in the chart below:

Above Diaphragm	Arm Channel	Element
Solid Organ	*related Hollow Organ*	
Heart	Small Intestine	Fire
Lung	Large Intestine	Wind
Pericardium	TriDosha (3D)	Water

Below Diaphragm	Leg Channel	Element
Solid Organ	*related Hollow Organ*	
Liver	Gallbladder	Ether
Spleen	Stomach	Earth
Kidney	Bladder	Water

CHANNELS-HUMORS CORRELATION

There is another very important reason why certain channels are positioned along the arm and yet others are found along the leg. This reason deals with the Ayurvedic concept of the three humors, Vata, Pitta and Kapha.

Along the arm, there must be a channel which directly deals with and affects Vata. Likewise, there must also be a channel which is related to Pitta and another to Kapha. Since there are six channels along the arm and six along the leg, there must be two channels which deal with each of the three humors. In other words, the solid and hollow organ channels found along a limb must mutually represent each of the three humors.

It is interesting to note that Charaka mentioned the whole body must receive Vata, Pitta and Kapha (in balanced proportions), since if this did not occur, no function or life would be present:

> "*Vata, Pitta and Kapha move all over the body; hence all the channels of the body cater to their needs for movement.*"[4]

HUMORAL CHANNELS IN ARM
Vata

Vata is represented in the arm by the Lung and Large Intestine channels, which are the solid and hollow Wind organs (Vata). These two organs are classified as primary Vata organs.

Pitta

Pitta is demonstrated by the organs which relate to Fire, a Pitta element, which are the Heart (solid organ) and the Small Intestine (hollow organ) channels. These two organs are classified as primary Pitta organs.

Kapha

Kapha in the arm is related to the organs, which are the pericardium (solid) and the Tridosha (hollow), since both of these organs deal with flow of fluids through the body. These are both Kapha related channels in the arm.

HUMORAL CHANNELS IN LEG

Vata

Vata is upheld in the leg by the Vata secondary type organs, which are the Kidney and the Bladder channels. These two have an undeniable connection with Vata since they are normally involved in Vata imbalances. These two organs have their channels along the leg.

Pitta

In the leg, Pitta is represented by the Liver and Gallbladder channels, both well-known Pitta organs. The channels are located in the leg to channel or control Pitta. The liver and gallbladder are considered secondary Pitta organs.

Kapha

In the leg, Kapha is represented by the Spleen (solid) and Stomach (hollow) organ channels due to Kapha's undeniable connection with Earth. In this case, these two are primary Kapha organs.

Inside-Outside Channels

The channels which relate to the solid organs, like the heart, liver, spleen, kidney and lung are located on the inside part of the limb, whether it is the leg or arm. The hollow organs, as in the large intestine, bladder, gallbladder, stomach and small intestine, have their channels along the outside of the arm or leg.

Ayurveda explains that the stomach, small intestine and large intestine (hollow organs) are readily available to the outside world. Food normally enters these organs before nutrients can reach the others.

Consequently, they are regarded as external organs and their channels are external channels. This means they are located on the outside of the limb (e.g back of the hand area of the arm). The solid ones are located on the inside area, e.g. the palm side of the arm.

OTHER PRANIC CHANNELS

In Ayurvedic Medicine and Yoga, there are literally thousands of minor nadi channels described. These connect with every structure of the body (including each cell) so as to supply the life energy, Prana, in order for living tissues to remain alive. Besides the channels which can be freely needled (acupunctured) to produce a therapeutic effect, there are others which perform various functions. These include the Ida, Sushumna and Surya channels.

Chakras

There are also major junctions of some channels (nadis) in the body which are called chakras.

Literally, chakra means "that which rotates" and essentially means a cycle or wheel. Chakras are energy fly-wheels found at various strategic locations. The chakras have their own types of channels, much like the acupuncture ones and are indeed related to them, yet separate.

There are seven major chakras in the body, five along the middle of the trunk and two on the head. There are also minor chakras at the wrists, elbows, ankles and knees (Figs. 3 & 4).

The five chakras located in the trunk are associated with the Five Elements in a direct relationship. The other two found in the head area are directly linked with Prana—the subtle bio-energy.

Interestingly, the order of appearance of the chakras is according to the Wheel of Creation, previously described, where each element follows another, according to their characteristics. It was explained that Prana occurs first, followed by Ether, Wind, Fire, Water and lastly Earth. The chakras too, follow this order.

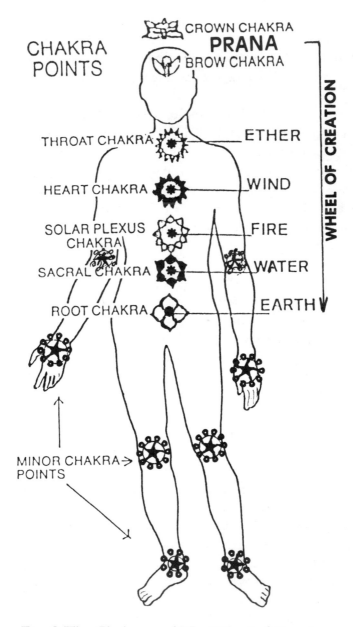

Fig. 3 The Chakras and The Wheel of Creation

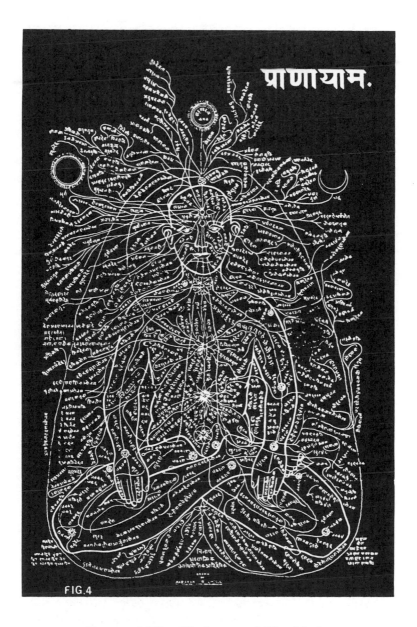

Figure 4 The Chakras and The Nadis

The chakras located on the head are found between the eyebrows and on the crown. They deal with intelligence, perception and the higher levels of the mind, a function of Prana.

Ajna Chakra
This is the so-called third eye located between the eyebrows. This chakra is the seat of the mind and usually relates to spiritual desires and aspirations. This is the site of Prana or primary energy of the body.

Sahasra Padma Chakra
This chakra is positioned in the middle of the crown and is interrelated to the third eye. Both deal with the intellect and upper levels of the mind. This is also the seat of Prana, as both of these chakras are joined.

Ether Chakra
The Ether chakra (Vissudhi) is found at the throat and sometimes is referred to as the Throat chakra. Like the Ether element, it is located at the first position along the Wheel of Creation, after Prana. Since Ether is the most subtle of the Five Elements, it is logical that this would be so. The Ether chakra contains Prana and consequently is related to Vata and its related types of diseases. This chakra is also related to the liver and gall bladder and can be involved in their dysfunctions.

Wind Chakra
The Wind chakra (Anahata) is positioned in the heart area (middle of both lungs) and is the seat of Wind. Consequently, it has an energetic connection to the lung and large intestine and is related to Wind dysfunctions.

Fire Chakra
The fire chakra (Manipura), or third chakra, is located down along the trunk. It is positioned in the navel area and physically relates to the small intestine and also the heart. It is energetically related to the

liver (via Pitta). Most Pitta humor dysfunctions are related to a malfunction in the Fire Chakra.

Water Chakra

The Water Chakra (Svadisthana) is the fourth and second to last chakra. It is positioned just above the sex organs and is related to the kidneys. Hence it also has a connection with the sexual system. Physiologically, the Water chakra is involved in Kapha syndromes as the source site of Water. Also this chakra has an effect on Vata and its type of dysfunctions, especially when there is a lack of Water in the body.

Earth Chakra

The Earth chakra (Muladhara) is found at the base of the spinal column and is the site of the element Earth. Physiologically, this chakra is involved in Vata problems since its position is in the Vata portion of the body. A lack of Earth can indeed result in a Vata disorder, as in anemia being a lack of iron (Earth substance). Energetically, this chakra also affects the spleen and stomach (and Kapha) as the source-site of the element Earth.

In reality, the three lower chakras (Fire, Water, Earth) are directly connected to dysfunctions of the three humors (Pitta, Vata and Kapha) due to their physical locations. On a subtle level, these also affect the organs which are energetically connected with them.

Treatment of imbalances of the elements can be applied to the area of the chakras. We may apply oils or even gems to these chakras to effect healing. Also, Acupuncture (Bhedankarma) and Moxibustion (Agnikarma) may be appropriate here.

Notes:

1. *Links Between Ayurveda and Acupuncture*, p. 5.
2. *Ibid.*, p. 9.
3. *Ayurveda—The Science of Self-Healing*, p. 56.
4. *Charaka Samhitta* V [6], p. 173.

CHAPTER IV

AYURVEDIC BIO-RHYTHMS
DISEASE RISK TIMES

Each humor or dosha has a specific time when it is most concentrated. It accumulates at specific times of the day, which in essence allows a humor in the body to be aggravated at that time. An established humoral dysfunction can then be made much worse during this time.

Each humor has four hours when it is most active, and can then demonstrate symptoms at that particular time. For instance, an imbalance of Vata can cause insomnia in the early hours of the morning. The patient may wake up at approximately 3-4 a.m. and then find it difficult to go back to sleep.

Each humor tends to increase, reaches a peak and then slowly decreases within a four hour span. A person with a humoral dysfunction, will find the symptoms worse during those four hours in which the humor's energy is greatest.

The renowned ancient Ayurvedic physician Charaka made it clear at what time of day or night we can expect to find humoral dysfunctions worse than others. Three thousand or more years ago, they understood the Ayurvedic Bio-rhythms. Charaka states:

> *"Specific time for the aggravation, manifestation of diseases is determined on the basis of the variations in seasons, timings of the day, night and intake of food."*[1]

He also stated the particular times of day when each humor can be unbalanced most and used the case of fever to illustrate these times:

> *"Vata fever: Occurrence or aggravation of fever after the digestion of food* **in the afternoon,** *[and]* **during dawn.**"[2]

This tends to point to Vata being worse in the afternoon—approximately from 3 p.m. to before dark (7 p.m.) and also before late morning (that is before 7 a.m.), during dawn.

*"Pitta fever: Simultaneous manifestation or aggravation of fever in the entire body, during the **mid-day**, [and] **midnight**."*[3]

Pitta can therefore be aggravated twice during a twenty four hour cycle, once during mid-day (11 a.m. - 3 p.m.) and also during midnight (11p.m. - 3a.m.).

*"Kapha fever: Simultaneous manifestation or aggravation of fever in the entire body, during the **fore-noon**, [and] **in the evening**."*[4]

It is obvious then that Charaka outlined the period before noon (no later than 11 a.m.) as the time of Kapha aggravation. He also mentioned the evening as another time of Kapha aggravation. This time is between the end of Vata time (7 p.m.) and the beginning of night Pitta time (11 p.m.). This similarly equates to four hours in which Kapha can be aggravated in the morning (before noon) and in the evening.

Accordingly, each humor may reflect its symptoms twice during a twenty-four hour cycle, for a length of four hours each. The Vata period in the early hours of the day (3 a.m. - 7 a.m.) has different type of (Vata) symptoms to the Vata in the afternoon (3 p.m. - 7 p.m.). In the morning, Vata is more powerful and deals with subtle problems like insomnia and nervousness, while in the afternoon it generally causes tiredness and exhaustion.

Pitta too has a superficial effect during noon as in skin rashes, while at night it demonstrates a deeper effect as in hyperacidity and ulcers. Kapha in the morning is greatly provoked while at night it liquifies.

ORGAN ENERGY PEAK

There is a reason why the humors tend to be more aggravated at specific times of the day or night. The humors tend to demonstrate dysfunctions at these times principally because of what occurs in their related organs.

Each organ is known to have two hours of greatest pranic activity. That is, Prana commences to increase, reaches a pinnacle or peak and then gradually decreases. All this occurs within two hours for the one organ. Prana then travels to the next organ in line, begins to increase, reaches a pinnacle and then decreases to then reach the next organ. This process continues ad infinitum. It is because of this increased pranic energy in the organ, that its related humor can be easily unbalanced. For instance, if Vata increases in the morning, this is normally due to a Vata organ increasing in energy at that time. This also applies for the other two humors—Pitta and Kapha.

Vata *(Wind)*
As mentioned by Charaka, Vata can be aggravated in the early morning. The lung and large intestine have already been explained as relating to the Wind element. It is the pranic energy peaking in these two organs at that time, that can cause Vata (wind) imbalances.

Kapha *(Earth)*
It is the Earth element -related organs of the stomach and spleen which next receive Prana after Vata. These two organs tend to peak prior to 11 a.m. (the start of Pitta). Charaka (XX) states that the *"Stomach and fat are the sites of Kapha".*[5] This results in an undeniable connection between this organ (stomach) and Kapha and its subsequent aggravation.

Pitta *(Fire)*
The heart and small intestine are the two Fire-related organs which have their energy peaking between 11 a.m. and 3 p.m., the hottest part of the day. It is then that Pitta dysfunctions tend to be more prevalent.
Charaka states that *"blood and the small intestine are the sites of Pitta."*[6] The heart and the small intestine are therefore totally involved here.

Vata *(deficient Water)*
The Vata related organs of the kidney and urinary bladder next receive Prana and begin to peak from 3 p.m. to 7 p.m., directly follow-

ing Pitta. Vata problems can then be highlighted at this time. Charaka once again enlightens us when he simply states that:

"The urinary bladder [and consequently the kidney] and colon are the sites of Vata."[7]

This points to the fact that not only the large intestine (colon) is a site for Vata, but also that the bladder (and kidney) are sites too.

Kapha *(Water)*

The organs of the pericardium and the Tridosha tend to affect Kapha in the evening between 7 p.m. and 11.p.m. These two will peak with Prana during this time so that Kapha will tend to liquify and cause Kapha-type symptoms.

Pitta *(Ether)*

The liver and gallbladder are Pitta organs according to Ayurveda. They come under the auspices of the Ether element. These two organs have pranic energy peaking between 11 p.m. and 3 a.m.

Dr. Vasant Lad explains that anger can affect Pitta and various Pitta-related organs:

"Repressed anger, for example completely changes the flora of the Gallbladder, bile duct and aggravates Pitta."[8]

It is obvious then, that Pitta, the gallbladder and the liver (which supplies bile through the duct) are interrelated and affected by anger, a Pitta negative emotion.

ENERGETICS BIO-RHYTHM CLOCK *(Pranic Mandala)*

The energetics bio-rhythm clock (Fig. 5) is one of the most useful tools in Ayurveda and particularly in Ayurvedic acupuncture. It provides a form of visualization which is necessary in the practice of acupuncture. Religiously taught in our college, the Australian Institute of Ayurvedic Medicine, the clock explains the undeniable connection between the various biological pranic systems including the humors and organs, pranic channels and times of most activity and risk. The

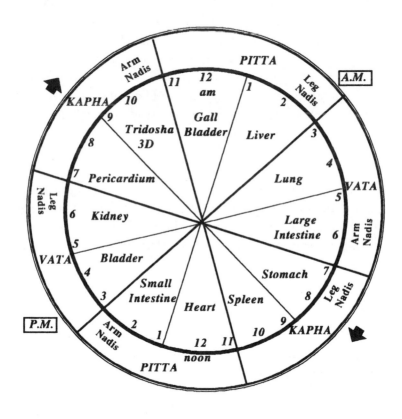

Fig. 5 The Pranic Mandala or Bio-Energy Clock

clock is also used in diagnosis, since an imbalance in a humor can be easily ascertained if the patient is able to tell what time of day (or night) his/her complaint appears worse. There is a strong correlation between the disease, the humoral imbalance and the related organ's energy peak.

Explanation

Each humor can be unbalanced twice in one day or a twenty-four hour cycle, once in the morning and once in the evening/night. This imbalance tends to be more prominent in a person of the same constitution as the humor which is unbalanced. Consequently, a Vata person with an established Vata dysfunction will feel worse during a Vata time (either in the early morning or in the afternoon). This also applies to the other two humors of Ayurveda (Kapha and Pitta).

The clock will then demonstrate which humor is unbalanced. It tells which organ or organs are related in the dysfunction and will ascertain the channel which can be needled in order to improve the humoral condition.

PRIMARY HUMORAL ORGANS

Each of the three humors has two Primary Organs, due to the direct effect and connection between them. The primary organs' energy peaks appear in the daytime (after 3 a.m. and before 3 p.m.—for 12 hours). The large intestine and lung are Vata primary organs not only because they are directly related to the element of Wind (an element of Vata), but also because the large intestine is the primary site of Vata.

Likewise, the stomach is the primary site of Kapha and due to its interrelation with the element of Earth, it forms one of the Kapha primary organs along with the spleen, its related solid organ.

The small intestine is the primary site of Pitta and consequently related to the element of Fire. By this connection, the S.I. is a primary Pitta organ along with the heart, which forms the connection via the blood, a Pitta tissue.

SECONDARY HUMORAL ORGANS

The secondary organs always appear after 3 p.m. and until 3 a.m. (for 12 hours). These organs connect with the humor via a secondary characteristic. These organs include the kidney and bladder for Vata, the liver and gallbladder for Pitta and the pericardium and the Tridosha for Kapha.

Each organ's position in the cycle or clock is according to a set pattern and does not change. This is due to the connection of the organs via their channels. Where a humor like Vata (in the a.m.) has two organs like the lungs and large intestine, their sequence of appearance in the cycle is permanent and according to established criteria. In the same humor, the two organs must not only be related but also must be of a solid and hollow type of connection. In the previous example of Vata, the solid organ is the lung, the hollow organ is the large intestine. When the humor changes from one to another as from Vata to Kapha in the morning, then the next organ along the line which receives Prana first must be the same type as the previous organ. In the case of Vata, since the large intestine was the last organ to receive Prana, then a similar type of Kapha organ must next be in line. In this case, the Kapha organ is the stomach, another hollow type of organ just like the large intestine. Subsequently, the spleen (a solid organ) receives Prana after the stomach and thus concluding Kapha in the morning (at 11 a.m.). This process continues for each twenty-four hour cycle. This is illustrated in the accompanying clock chart (Pranic Mandala—Fig. 5).

VATA (a.m.)	3 - 5 a.m.	Lung (solid organ)
(Arm channels)	5 - 7 a.m.	Large Intestine (hollow organ)
KAPHA	7 - 9 a.m.	Stomach (hollow organ)
(Leg channels)	9 - 11 a.m.	Spleen (solid organ)
PITTA	11 a.m. - 1 p.m.	Heart (solid organ)
(Arm channels)	1 p.m. - 3 p.m.	Small Intestine (hollow organ)

VATA (p.m.)	3 - 5 p.m.	Urinary Bladder (hollow organ)
(Leg channels)	5 - 7 p.m.	Kidney (solid organ)
KAPHA	7 - 9 p.m.	Pericardium (solid organ)
(Arm channels)	9 - 11 p.m.	Tridosha (hollow organ)
PITTA	11 p.m. - 1 a.m.	Gallbladder (hollow organ)
(Leg channels)	1 a.m. - 3 a.m.	Liver (solid organ)

One of the interesting things about the above concept is that the organ channels (nadis) connect with each other according to the above scheme and carry Prana according to the times and method above. For instance, the Heart channel connects with the Small Intestine channel which then connects with the Urinary Bladder channel, then the Kidney channel, etc.

Another very important point about the above concept is that each humor has its organ channels on the one limb (e.g. arm). The subsequent humor has its channels on the opposing limb (e.g. leg) and the following one after that, has its channels back on the arm again. This process continues in the same format until all the channels have been covered.

The pranic flow through the channels is also according to the above scheme, in the form of a loop.

THE AYURVEDIC ENERGY WHEELS

Ayurveda explains that there is a sequence of creation of the Five Elements and consequently the humors. Humors and elements lead in a cyclic manner in order for life to emerge, to continue and to finally decay. This is primarily due to the flow of Prana through the channels, and secondarily to the flow of the humors throughout the body.

Charaka explains that not only is there a wheel of creation but also one of destruction, since the latter relates to how living beings finally perish.

"The Universe moves around from the unmanifested stage to the manifested one [Creation] and then again from the manifested stage to the unmanifested one [Destruction]."[9]

It is absolutely necessary to realize that according to classical Ayurveda, the Five Elements appeared in a specific order, so as to form the cosmos. This primordial order which we call a cycle or wheel is the basis on which other cycles or wheels of the body are based. This Wheel of Creation (Nirmana Chakra) and its three derivative wheels describe the major functions of the body. Consequently, there must be a creating, a controlling, a destroying and a supporting function. These are the four natural functions which form and affect homeostasis (health). The Creation Wheel describes the birth process; the Supporting Wheel describes how we continue to survive; the Controlling Wheel describes the mechanism by which the body keeps itself from "going over the top"; and the Destruction Wheel describes the method by which we finally die.

This can be compared to an automobile—

CREATION—vehicle assembled at the automobile plant

SUPPORTING—Accelerator pedal / gas, oil and water

CONTROLLING—Brake pedal/hand brake

DESTRUCTION—Wear and tear, non-service of vehicle, accident

There are another two cycles which evolve from creation and together compose the processes of creation, controlling, destroying and supporting functions. All these functions are qualities of Prana, the first energy.

Renown Yoga master and author of *Light on Pranayama*, B.K.S. Iyengar, describes Prana's functions as follows:

"Prana is energy which creates, protects and destroys."[10]

These are the natural functions which form life and affect homeostasis (health).

Creation

The Wheel of Creation describes the birth process, creation, and how Prana develops from pure energy into the most physical of its forms in the body.

Protection

Protection is offered by the Wheel of Support which describes how processes continue to function, one element feeding the next. The Wheel of Control describes the mechanisms by which the body keeps itself from 'going over the top' with regard to the Elements. Both the Supporting and Controlling Wheels are forms of protection.

Destruction

The Wheel of Destruction describes the method by which diseases occur and how we finally become ill and consequently die.

This can be compared to an automobile: Creation—vehicle assembled at the automobile factory. Supporting—accelerator pedal/gas, oil and water. Controlling—brake pedal, hand brake and steering wheel. Destruction—wear and tear, prolonged non-service of vehicle, collisions.

WHEEL OF CREATION (Nirmana Chakra)

The sequence of the creation of the five physical elements (Panchamahabhutas) was previously described as the Wheel of Creation (see Fig. 6). Each element in the cycle helped to create the next one in line, from most subtle to most physical. Prana, the life energy, was the most subtle of all which preceded the five. Their progressive development also allowed the creation of the three humors in the order of most subtle effect, that is Vata, Pitta and lastly Kapha.

Ether + Wind = Vata
Fire + Water = Pitta
Water + Earth = Kapha

The Wheel of Creation is related to Kapha, the anabolic (building-up) humor in the body.

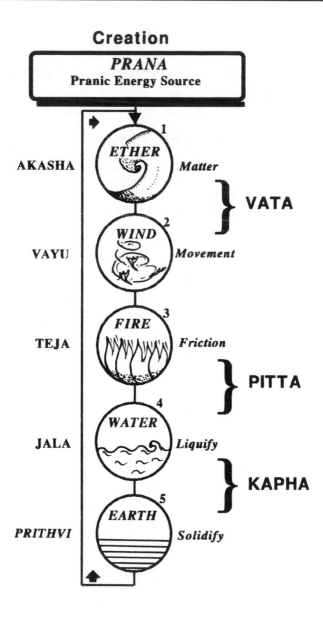

Fig. 6 Wheel of Creation—Nirmana-Chakra
Prana and the Five Elements interaction

WHEEL OF DESTRUCTION *(Vinasha Chakra)*

Upon formation via the previously mentioned wheel, the body then begins a slow trek towards its own physical destruction, through gradual decay so that the elements and Prana can return back to their source. This process may take anywhere from birth to about 110 years of age.

Ayurveda also points out that we as humans go through three stages of life, resembling the three humors.

1. Kapha stage—childhood to adolescent (1-14 yrs.)

2. Pitta stage—adolescent to adulthood (15-45 yrs.)

3. Vata stage—middle age to old age (45+ yrs.)

Kapha during childhood normally involves respiratory dysfunctions e.g. congestion and Kapha type syndromes.

The Pitta stage involves digestive disorders.

Vata being the last stage deals with Vata type syndromes, like wrinkles, dry skin and bones (osteoporosis), etc. It virtually dries out the body.

The Wheel of Destruction (Fig. 7) is the process by which the body decays. This means that the dysfunctions start in subtle problems— (Vata), and later reach the most serious form—the most physical in malady (Kapha). Consequently, the elements also occur in said manner, where the cycle involves Ether first then Wind (Vata), Fire and Water (Pitta), and lastly Earth (Kapha). This is exemplified in Ayurveda by Charaka who cites that Vata is responsible for more diseases than Pitta or Kapha. In fact, the ratio is 80 Vata: 40 Pitta: 20 Kapha.

As the illness begins in an imbalance of Prana and Vata (subtle) until it reaches its most physical form, so the sequence of decay similarly occurs in this way. A chronic disease has reached its most physical form (Kapha) from its most acute imbalance (Vata).

The Wheel of Destruction can be used to identify the process of illness by determining which organs are affected, according to this cycle. The elements can destroy each other in the following manner. The Wheel of Destruction is analogous to Vata, the catabolic humor.

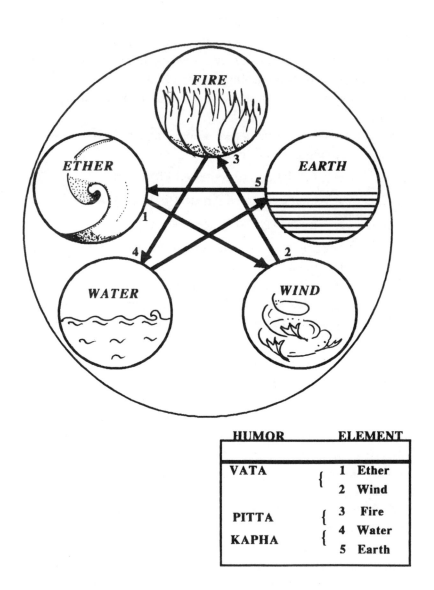

HUMOR	ELEMENT
VATA {	1 Ether
	2 Wind
PITTA {	3 Fire
KAPHA {	4 Water
	5 Earth

Fig. 7 Wheel of Destruction *(Vinasha Chakra)*

Ether-Wind

The quality of Ether in the body is usually one of heat since this relates to the liver, gallbladder and Pitta. Consequently, Ether can destroy Wind by overheating it, causing dryness (as in a desert) and aggravating Vata, as well as the nervous system, due to excess heat.

Wind-Fire

Wind can destroy Fire by blowing it out, when in excess. This is like blowing out a candle. Excess Wind destroys Fire through increasing nervousness by destroying the balance of the heart which controls the nerves. Also, Wind as in excess Vata can reduce Agni, the digestive fire in the small intestine (a Fire organ as well). Also, a long term smoker may experience heart disease (increase in blood pressure etc.) due to the increase in Wind (smoke).

Fire-Water

Excess Fire as in high Pitta can destroy Water in the body by overheating and causing dehydration. This is similar to a high fever, and its resultant great thirst.

Water-Earth

Water can similarly destroy Earth as the feature of Earth is rigidity, solidity and lack of movement. Water in excess can cause fluid retention. This would unlock Earth's rigid grip on the muscles etc. by allowing unwanted movement (as in loose joints, swollen ankles etc.). This would result in a high Kapha syndrome. Balanced Water and Earth is essential for normal Kapha.

Earth-Ether

The quality of Earth is coldness which is also a quality of Kapha. Through this excess coldness, Earth can destroy the heat of Ether in the liver, a Pitta organ.

The Wheel of Destruction resembles Vata and its catabolic (destructive) effect. This wheel is also called the wheel of dissolution and as Feuerstein explains:

> "*The process is described in the* Mahanirvana-Tantra *(V.93ff.). According to this passage, the process of dissolution is as follows: the element earth is dissolved into that of water, water into fire, fire into air, air into ether, ether into the sense of egoity... into the world ground and... into the transcendent.*"[11]

THE WHEEL OF CONTROL *(Vinaya Chakra)*

Each element due to its interconnection via a subtle channel with organs and humors, also undergoes a sequence of control. The controlling action represents a damper or brake on the element's action, so that the elements remain at a correct level or equilibrium. When an element fails to control its corresponding element, the latter one will tend to malfunction in accordance with its attributes. For instance, if Ether fails to control Earth, then rigidity, heaviness and lack of appetite may set in. This is characteristic of a dysfunctional Kapha. In this case, Ether can not prevent Kapha's negative attributes from increasing.

The controlling function is extremely important. Without proper control, each element would tend to go on its own way, increasing in accordance with its inherent quality, without a safety brake.

The Wheel of Control (Fig. 8) is related to Pitta, the metabolic or regulating humor. The elements control each other in the following manner:
1. Ether controls Earth.
2. Earth controls Water.
3. Water controls Fire.
4. Fire controls Wind.
5. Wind controls Ether.

THE WHEEL OF SUPPORT *(Alamba Chakra)*

The Alambachakra or Wheel of Support (Fig. 10) occurs when each element supports the next one in line, by handing over its pranic

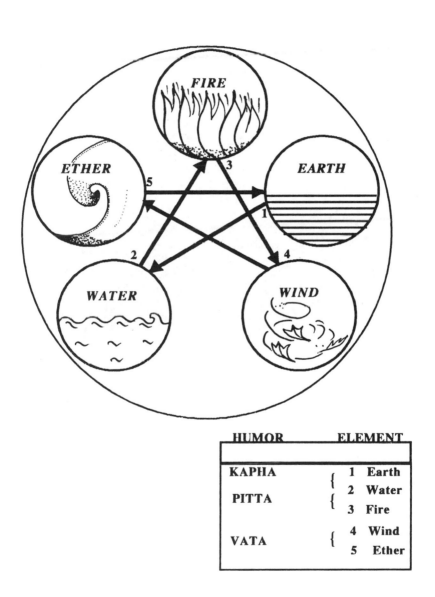

Fig. 8 The Wheel of Control *(Vinaya Chakra)*

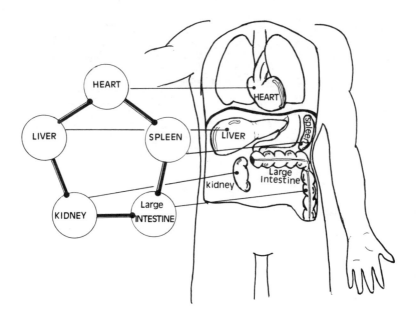

Fig. 9 Anatomical position of the organs in the body and in the Wheels

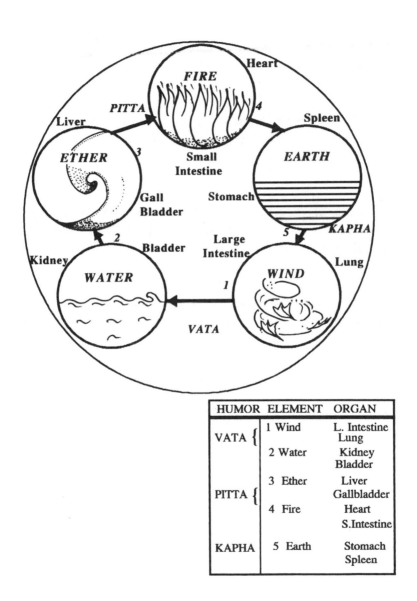

HUMOR	ELEMENT	ORGAN
VATA {	1 Wind	L. Intestine Lung
	2 Water	Kidney Bladder
PITTA {	3 Ether	Liver Gallbladder
	4 Fire	Heart S.Intestine
KAPHA	5 Earth	Stomach Spleen

Fig. 10 The Wheel of Support *Alamba Chakra)*

energy. This is similar to the way a mother breast feeds her child. Without the support obtained from food the child would perish. The support differs from control in that a child may be fed by the mother (support) but is taught by the teacher (control). In most cases, the teacher and parent are two different people.

This sequence of support is similar to that of Creation where Vata leads to Pitta which finally leads to Kapha. However, this support concerns the organs so that they appear according to the appearance of the three humors.

Vata

In the case of Vata, the large intestine and lung appear for Wind, while the kidney and urinary bladder appear for Vata but under the Water element.

Pitta

In the case of Pitta, the liver and gallbladder appear via the Ether element, while the heart and small intestine appear under Fire.

Kapha

In the case of Kapha, the spleen and stomach appear under the Earth element.

This is then the order of appearance of the organs:

Wind	Large Intestine	**Vata**
	Lung	
Water	Kidney	
	Bladder	
Ether	Liver	**Pitta**
	Gallbladder	
Fire	Heart	
	Small Intestine	
Earth	Spleen	**Kapha**
	Stomach	

WHEELS INTERACTIONS

Where a dysfunction occurs, several of the wheels described above will become involved.

In the event that an element became in excess due to a number of factors including stress, incorrect food, seasonal changes, etc., this would follow a certain path. The excess element would tend to over-control its related element (according to the Wheel of Control) and destroy the other (according to the Wheel of Destruction). For instance, if Ether (Pitta) became in excess (see Fig. 11) due to excessive anger (a Pitta emotion), it may tend to over-control Earth (Kapha) which may cause a lack of appetite and destroy (attack) Wind (Vata). In the latter, excessive heat can over-stimulate Vata and cause it to flare up.

This concept is applicable to the other elements as follows:

Excess

Fire *(Pitta)*

When Fire is in excess, this relates to high Pitta which automatically reduces Kapha (destroy Water) and over-controls Vata (over-control Wind).

Earth *(Kapha)*

When Earth is in excess, this equates to high Kapha (rigidity, obesity). This results in restriction of Water in the body due to the excess earth (over-control of Water) and destroys Ether, which in this case relates to Pitta or heat, since the cold effect of Earth cools down the heat.

Wind *(Vata)*

When Wind is in excess, this equals high Vata, so that Fire is destroyed (Vata would perhaps attack the blood—RaktaVata). The cold effect of Wind also lowers the fire of Pitta via the Ether (over-controlling it).

Water *(Kapha)*

When Water is in excess, this results in high Kapha (of excess fluid).

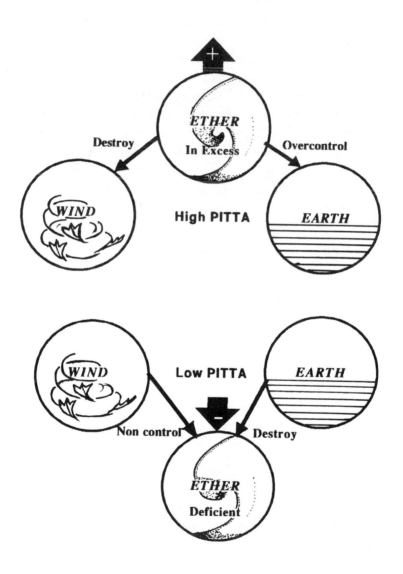

Fig. 11 Elements' Excesses and Deficiencies

Consequently, this Kapha lowers Pitta (over-control Fire), and at the same time destroys Earth (excess water added to a bucket of earth destroys the effect of earth and cause looseness, etc.).

Ether *(Pitta)*
When Ether is in excess, this normally causes a high Pitta condition as in excess energy in the liver and gallbladder. The result is a lowering of Kapha (cold) by over-controlling Earth. At the same time, the drying effect of ether (dry heat) combined with excess heat destroys (attacks) Wind or Vata. Excess dry heat obviously over-stimulates or aggravates Vata.

Deficiency
In cases of element (or humor) deficiency, the other elements (or humors) tend to attack the weakened element. Consequently, when Fire (Pitta) is deficient, both Vata and Kapha attack it. This means that Water attacks Fire (Kapha reduces Pitta) and Vata also affects it. Wind's cold and windy effect may put out the fire.

Fire
Fire/Pitta low , Kapha high (Water), Vata high (Wind).

Ether
Ether/Pitta low, Kapha high (Earth), Vata high (Wind).

Earth
Earth/Kapha low, Pitta high (Ether), Vata high (Water low)

Wind
Wind/Vata low, Pitta high (heat and moisture) both Ether and Fire. If Vata is low, then Pitta must be high (more oiliness or moisture).

WHEEL OF THE TISSUES
Ayurveda states that there are seven types of tissues in the human body. These tissues called Dhatus are the physical sphere in which the humors develop and the physical site of their imbalance. Essen-

tially, every organ and system is made up of at least one of these tissues. Hence, the later development of disease in the organs can occur through the elements, humors and tissues.

Traditionally, Ayurveda outlines seven types of tissues. They appear in the following descending order and actually form a loop or cycle. This cycle is called DhatuChakra or the Wheel of the Tissues:

1. Plasma
2. Blood
3. Muscle
4. Fat
5. Bone
6. Marrow and nerves
7. Reproductive tissue

Many reasons have been cited in the past for the mutual connection of the seven tissues. Three major reasons are explained.

The first relates to one tissue turning itself into another. It is difficult to understand how muscle can turn into fat (science believes this is not possible).

The second says that some tissues irrigate others as in blood irrigating muscle. This tends to be incomplete.

The third, more modern idea, relates to communication between tissues via hormones or enzymes to trigger a reaction.

The so-called one tissue creating another tissue is more correctly explained as one tissue "nourishing" another tissue. Since Prana is the essence or energy of life, then this communication is via Prana. The communication mirrors the way that Prana communicates and "nourishes" each organ, according to the Five Elements (Fig. 12). This effect is via an energetic connection and interrelated to pranic flow through the channels (especially the Nadis). Sharma and Dash in the *Charaka* (Vol.II) explain it in the following manner:

"So dhatus [tissues] are nourished through their respective channels and one channel cannot provide nourishment to another dhatu as one canal cannot irrigate trees situated in different places (directions) [unless it is done via its respective, dedicated dhatu channel]."[12]

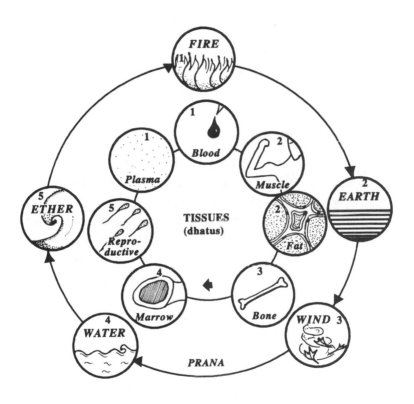

Fig. 12 The Wheel of the Tissues *(Dhatu Chakra)*

Since Prana is the essential energy which keeps everything alive and healthy, the dhatus or tissues communicate with each other via the Pranic channels. This is reminiscent of the way each element supports (or feeds) each other according to the Wheel of Support, described earlier.

The only problem that appears to arise in this meshing of the elements and the tissues is that there are five elements and seven tissues. It is difficult to see how they integrate since their numbers are different.

The Wheel of Support relates the elements in a cyclic manner but each element supports one another according to the following scheme: Fire, Earth, Wind, Water and Ether. After Ether, Fire then commences once again in a loop form.

FIRE

"Plasma [rasa] and blood [rakta] are the sites of Pitta [fire]" [13]

Ayurveda then agrees that both of these tissues are related to the Fire element and Pitta. Plasma (rasa) is the watery substance in blood containing food nutrients primarily received from and absorbed through the small intestine. Plasma then has a connection with Fire, since the small intestine is a Fire organ. Blood (rakta) carries oxygen, etc. to all tissues. Blood is composed of the Fire and Water elements (Pitta). Blood is then related to this humor and is pumped through the body by the heart (another Fire organ).

EARTH

Muscle and fat both relate to Earth. The spleen (pancreas) and stomach relate to these two tissues through their Earth connection. Charaka once again deciphers this when he states the connection of fat, muscle and Kapha (which is related to Earth): *"Due to the vitiation of Kapha. Obesity [fat, and] loss of strength [muscle deficiency]."* [14]

Muscle, through the pranic energy of the spleen and its channel nourishes Fat (pancreas). Charaka agrees that diabetes, a pancreatic disorder, is caused by the vitiation of fat. [15] So the connection of the pancreas to the Earth element and fat is obvious.

By muscle and fat's interconnection with the Earth element (the element of growth), the tissues are reduced to five in number, according to the Five Elements.

WIND
Bone relates to Wind and Vata. Dr. Vasant Lad explains this when he states that *"The Large Intestine and bones are the seats of Vata."*[16]

The large intestine and lungs, both of Wind origin, have a direct effect and relationship to Bone. The previous energy in Earth is fed to Wind (Bone) for nourishment.

WATER
Marrow relates to Water, yet it is also considered a Vata tissue since vitiation of Marrow aggravates Vata and the nerves. Since the kidneys and its related organ, the urinary bladder, affect Vata, Water is related to Vata, kidneys and bladder and Marrow. Charaka states that the bladder [and kidney] is the site of Vata. [17] The energy from the Wind is fed to Water to nourish the kidneys and marrow.

ETHER
Reproductive tissue relates to Ether. This is because *"the fruit [reproductive tissue] corresponds to Ether, the subtle essence of the plant."*[18]

The human fruit (that which enables reproduction) is akin to the plant's fruit and similarly related to the Ether element. Consequently, the liver and gallbladder are Ether organs and related to the reproductive tissue.

The seven tissues, which can be reduced down to five due to their mutual interactions (e.g. muscle/fat and plasma/blood), mimic the Five elements in the Wheel of Support.

WHEEL OF SUPPORT

Tissue	Element	Humor
Plasma/Blood	Fire	Pitta
Muscle/Fat	Earth	Kapha
Bone	Wind	Vata
Marrow	Water	Vata
Reproductive	Ether	Pitta (+Vata+Kapha)

The sequence of the tissues nourishing or feeding one another via their respective channels is called DhatuChakra. This wheel is identical to the Wheel of Support and consequently, imbalances in the tissues can be treated with acupuncture by treating the appropriate channels and points related to the Five Elements. Their essence in common and their communication is through Prana, the life energy.

Notes:

1. *Charaka Samhitta*, p. 14.
2. *Ibid.*, p. 20
3. *Ibid.*, pp. 21-22.
4. *Ibid.*, p. 24.
5. *Ibid.*, p. 362.
6. *Ibid.*, p. 362.
7. *Ibid.*, p. 362.
8. *Ayurveda—The Science of Self-Healing*, p. 40.
9. *Charaka Samhitta*, Sarirasthana I [67-69], p. 328.
10. *Light on Pranayama*, p. 12.
11. *Textbook of Yoga*, p. 155.
12. *Charaka Samhitta*, p. 172.
13. *Ibid.*, Vol. I, p. 362.
14. *Ibid.*, Vol 1, p. 370.
15. *Ibid.*, p. 577.
16. *Ayurveda—The Science of Self-Healing*, p. 30.
17. *Charaka*, p. 362.
18. *Yoga of Herbs*, p. 10.

CHAPTER V

PART 1

MAJOR ORGANS

There are two types of internal major organs in the human body according to Ayurveda. Some organs are considered solid because for all intent and purposes they are solid, at least more solid than others. They are also very necessary and normally cannot be removed by surgery. For instance, the heart is a solid organ and cannot be removed without the person dying. This also applies to others like the liver or even the kidneys. Even though humans have two kidneys and can survive with only one, if both are removed, the person will die.

The other type of organs are referred to as hollow, since they do, in most cases, resemble a hollow pipe or sack, e.g. the large and small intestines and the stomach. Hollow organs are necessary for the correct function of the body, however they can often be removed without the person dying (e.g. gallbladder, part of the colon etc.). The digestive tract organs, hollow organs, are considered very important in Ayurveda, since it is there that Vata, Pitta and Kapha dysfunctions first originate and later migrate to other parts of the body.

There are six solid and six hollow organs classified in Ayurveda.

FUNCTIONS OF THE SIX SOLID ORGANS

(1) Heart

The heart controls the flow of blood through the body and is the site of Prana, which often controls mental activity according to Charaka. The heart is responsible for the health of the blood vessels. Physiologically, the heart is an involuntary muscle which acts as a pump, contracting and expanding to force blood to all parts of the body. The heart consists of four separate chambers, the upper two are called the Atria (left and right) while the lower two are called the Ventricles. These compartments are separated by muscular partitions called septa (singular: septum). There are also four valves which regulate the flow of blood, two semilunar valves, one tricuspid and one bicuspid or mitral valves.

The heart is related to Kapha because it is essentially made of muscle (Earth), but also it is energetically connected to Pitta and the Fire element as well, through its connection with blood. The heart has a pranic channel (nadi) which commences in the heart. It is then logically called the Heart channel.

(2) Lung

The lung controls the flow of water and Prana through the body. This occurs because it is only by Prana flowing correctly through the channels that water (body fluids) can similarly flow.

It is responsible for the health of the skin and hair, since being a Vata organ it relates to the Wind element. There are two lungs in the body, one on the right side and one on the left side of the body. Oxygen which carries Prana is taken into the blood and then diffused into the blood stream to be carried elsewhere. Waste carbon dioxide is excreted from the body via the lungs and expiration.

(3) Liver

The liver is positioned in the right hypochondria (under the breathing diaphragm).It controls the unobstruction of Prana and blood, and is responsible for the health of the tendons due to their connection with Pitta. The liver also receives food nutrients from the stomach and intestines via the portal veins. It produces and stores various vitamins, sugars and minerals. It also digests the Five Elements (e.g. from a vegetable) and turns them into the form which can be used by the body. This is achieved by the Bhuta-Agnis, the five liver fires which digest the elements. The liver is a Pitta organ, since the word *pitta* itself is translated as *bile*, a product which is produced by the liver.

(4) Spleen

The spleen controls digestion and the transportation of blood. It is responsible for the muscles. The spleen, positioned in the upper left side of the abdominal cavity, functions also to remove and destroy disease-producing organisms from the blood stream. It stores blood in order to release it when required, as when excessive bleeding occurs. Due to its connection with the blood, the spleen is related to Pitta. However, it is also related to Kapha because of its connection with the earth element and its attribute of growth. In fact, the difference between muscle and fat (both contain earth and water) is that the spleen heavily deals with blood, and through its heat (fire) it turns earth and water (as though by baking) into muscle. It is the heat that makes the difference between muscle and fat. Fat is analogous to gelatin powder (earth) and water; it results in a cold, unstable (floppy) concoction. Muscle, on the other hand, is like making a mixture of cake powder (earth) and water and placing it in the oven (heat) to bake. The result is like a solid structure, much more stable than the gelatin (jelly) product. The spleen has a pranic channel which connects with the legs.

(5) Kidney

The two kidneys are positioned directly behind the eighth to tenth ribs. It controls water metabolism and is responsible for the bones, marrow and affects the reproductive organs since these are positioned in the Vata area of the trunk. It also separates waste products and water from the blood to excrete as urine. Through its drying action on fluids in the body (just like a flood-gate), the kidneys relate to Vata. When it removes water, it relates to Vata, but while it retains water in the body, it deals with Kapha. The kidney has a pranic channel which connects with the legs.

(6) Pericardium

Although not strictly an organ per se, the pericardium is nevertheless recognized as one in Ayurveda. It is a sac which surrounds the heart and usually swells with fluid during a disease (pericarditis). It is connected to the diaphragm, the heart blood vessels and the thoracic wall. This organ has an effect on the Kapha flow. Its pranic energy channel is located along the arms.

FUNCTIONS OF THE SIX HOLLOW ORGANS

(1) Stomach

The stomach is positioned in the upper part of the abdominal cavity. It is connected with the esophagus at the top end and at the small intestine by the pyloric sphincter or valve. Its main function is to receive and macerate food with the aid of the gastric juices. This mixture is eventually thinned down into chyme which exits the stomach and enters the duodenum (small intestine). Some experts believe that it is a subtle form of chyme which is produced in the stomach and attacks the lung when Kapha is aggravated.

The stomach works in conjunction with the spleen which carries on the functions of digestion and absorption. As with the spleen, with which it is internally related, the stomach also affects the muscles. Growth in the body is under the control of Kapha, the anabolic humor. The stomach is a very important part of this humor. The Stomach channel is positioned along the legs in a direct relationship with the spleen.

(2) Large Intestine

The large intestine consists of four sections, the cecum, ascending, transverse and descending colons and is approximately five feet in length. The large intestine absorbs moisture from the digested food, and is also extremely important in the absorption of Prana from food into the body. It manufactures some vitamins in the intestinal flora, forms feces and expels them by the use of peristalsis (waves).

The large intestine is related to Vata and Wind, and consequently to the lungs and also has an effect on the skin and hair. The Large Intestine channel is located along the arm in a relative position to the Lung channel.

(3) Small Intestine

The small intestine is positioned in the abdominal area and absorbs 90% of all nutrients. It is approximately twenty feet in length. Since the small intestine is a Fire organ and is related to the heart with which it is internally connected, it is also involved in the health of the blood vessels. The small intestine is also the site of Agni, the digestive fire.

When Agni becomes low (which can occur due to antibiotics, stress etc.) the digestive process will falter, causing malabsorption of nutrients and the consequential effect of Ama, or toxin build-up in the body. Also, due to low Agni (fire) in the small intestine, various germs and mold, etc. (e.g. candida) can be allowed a safe passage to the large intestine where they lodge and begin to cause dysfunctions.

The Small Intestine channel is located in the arm in a relative position to the Heart channel, with which it is related.

(4) Gallbladder

The gallbladder, a sack-like structure, stores bile (greenish fluid) which is produced by the liver and used in the digestive process. The Gallbladder channel is connected with the Liver channel and is also responsible for the unobstruction of Prana as well as the health of the tendons. The gallbladder, due to its connection with the liver, is directly connected to the Ether element and to Pitta.

(5) Urinary Bladder

The urinary bladder is a membranous sack which stores urine after it is produced and excreted by the kidneys. It connects with the kidneys via two pipes called ureters. The bladder and the kidneys both affect the health of the bones, marrow and the reproductive system, related to Vata.

(6) Tridosha (3D)

The tridosha is not a physiological organ per se, but in Ayurveda it is considered as such. Tridosha is a generalization of the three areas of the trunk which relate to the three humors (doshas). These are Vata, Pitta and Kapha.

As the trunk can be considered a hollow pipe, then the Tridosha is a hollow organ. Tridoshas literally means "three-humors". The flow of fluids through these three areas of the trunk can be affected by an imbalance in one or more of the three humors, so that the mutual balance of all is reflected in the Tridosha and its pranic channel. The Tridosha (3D) and the pericardium are therefore related and their pranic channels interconnect.

PART 2

THE TWO OPPOSITES *(Guna Dvandva)*

There is a theory of opposite and interdependent qualities, objects and forces in the universe, according to Ayurveda.

These forces are continuous, active polarities which affect all of the animate world. Both of these types of forces are in conflict yet interdependent and through this, things live and flourish. Through their conflict, things deteriorate and die. Both phases are important parts of Life.

These opposing yet related and inter-dependent forces are called Guna-Dvandva which literally means "qualities of duality". It is because of Prana-life energy that everything exists, but it is through Akasha (Ether) that things are allowed to take shape, since Ether is the field (or matrix) on which everything is created. Prana (energy) therefore relies on Ether (matter) for life to exist, yet they are both opposite forces. Due to the qualities of the Five Elements, every object has a prominence of a particular quality in accordance to the attributes of the element.

Essentially, everything in the universe can be classified and divided into two such groups, each requiring the other for survival. Life, for instance, acting as the rising and falling curve of a sine wave, supplies us with many moments which are extremely joyous and happy. Later, we may take delivery of a most horrendous shipment of sorrow. Both aspects are part of life and we must learn to handle them and learn from them, to avoid complications. Someone once said that "there is no such thing as problems, only opportunities." We must learn to "ride the wave."

As the Buddha reportedly said, "the measure of a real person is not one who never falls, but rather when the person does fall, he/she gets up again."

The Sun and the Moon are also of these opposite polarities. Solar energy is positive energy, while Lunar energy is negative, yet we are dependent on both for our existence. Without males, humans cannot reproduce, without females, they would also be in great difficulty.

All energies and matter have definite attributes (gunas). All objects normally have more than one characteristic or property and can be recognized by their relationship to duality (dvandva).

The ancient Ayurvedic physician Charaka wrote a commentary on the attributes or dual qualities. He outlined ten pairs of such attributes as found in Nature. But he did so not to illustrate that there are only ten pairs, but rather that the ones mentioned below form an effective part of Ayurvedic diagnosis and treatment.[1] These ten paired sets of qualities are extremely important. Charaka states: *"The twenty qualities . . .are useful for [various] therapies."*[2] Sharma and Dash comment further: *"Attributes like superiority and inferiority are not relevant from the standpoint of treatment; hence they are not described here [by Charaka]."*[3]

It is obvious that Charaka needed to describe these important qualities of duality for diagnosis and therapy, but that he did not need to describe others which he was totally aware of, such as, dark and light, left and right, Sun and Moon, male and female, etc.

He listed and described the following twenty (ten pairs of interrelated attributes):

1. (a) Heavy (guru)   (b) Light (laghu)
2. (a) Cold (sita)   (b) Hot (ushna)
3. (a) Oily (snigdha)   (b) Dry (ruksa)
4. (a) Slow (manda)   (b) Quick (tiksna)
5. (a) Static (sthira)   (b) Mobile (sara)
6. (a) Soft (mrdu)   (b) Hard (kathina)
7. (a) Clear (vishada)   (b) Turbid (picchila)

8. (a) Smooth (slakshna)   (b) Rough (khara)
9. (a) Gross (sthula)   (b) Subtle (suksma)
10. (a) Solid (sandra)   (b) Liquid (drava)

Ayurveda, literally being the "Science of Life," is aware of and takes into account all qualities of an opposite nature, and not just the ten pairs outlined above.

We should not be blinded by the fact that there exist three humors and five elements. The concept of duality is still applicable to all of them. The Gunas have their particular properties or attributes due to their interconnection with the Five Elements. A *heavy* quality (1a), for instance, is weight increasing and consequently not only relates to Water and Earth but to Kapha as well. The *light* quality (1b), on the other hand, being weight reducing is found in the Fire, Wind and Ether elements and in Pitta and Vata. Any substance which has one of these attributes must have a link with at least one of the Five Elements. Where there is dry skin (3b), oil may be therapeutic (3a).

GUNAS	ELEMENT
Heavy	Earth/Water
Light	Fire/Wind/Ether
Cold	Water/Earth
Hot	Fire/Ether (Pitta)
Oily	Water
Dry	Earth/Fire/Wind/Ether
Slow	Earth/Water
Quick	Fire
Static	Earth
Mobile	Wind
Soft	Water/Ether
Hard	Earth

Clear	Wind/Fire/Ether
Turbid	Water/Earth
Smooth	Fire
Rough	Wind
Gross	Earth
Subtle	Ether/Wind/Fire
Solid	Earth
Liquid	Water

Left—Right

Ayurveda classifies the body as being divided into two opposite but interdependent halves, that is a left and a right half. The left half, under the control of Ida Nadi (channel), is usually cool. The right half, under the control of the Surya Nadi (Sun Channel), is usually warm (Fig. 13). Of course, the difference in temperature between one side and the other is not normally noticeable.

The Ida channel originates in the left nostril and is influenced by Lunar energy which has a cold attribute. Charaka himself stated this: *"The Moon is the presiding deity [force] of Water. The water in the atmosphere (before it falls on the ground) is by nature cold."*⁴

This channel allows cool air to enter the body.

The Surya (or Pingala) channel, on the other hand, is influenced by the Sun and has a hot quality. The channel originates in the right nostril and allows warm air to enter the body.

The left side of the body is related to negative energy which has Kapha and Vata properties. Consequently, many of the types of diseases related to these two humors affect the left side of the body. Also, since a female is directly related to the Kapha/Vata humors, she is also under the influence of the Moon, just as Water is.

The right side of the body relates to positive energy which has Pitta qualities. Many Pitta type diseases affect the male, (who is more Pitta than the female) and the right side of the body.

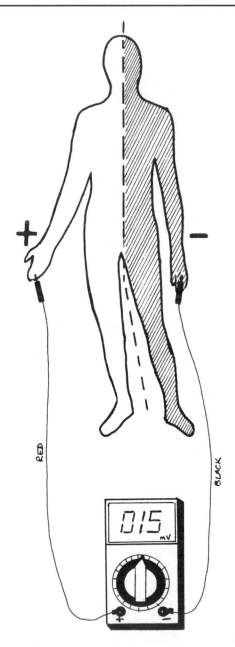

Fig. 13 The Right and Left Sides (Pitta & Kapha) and polarities

The Spleen, being a Kapha organ, has a physical effect on the left side of the body and Kapha. The liver, being related to Pitta, has a similar effect on the actions of Pitta. When a person lies down on one side of the body, this tends to suppress one of the two organs mentioned above and allows the other side, controlled by the opposite organ to increase its qualities. For example, when lying down on the right side, this would suppress the function of the liver (and Pitta), which would then allow the spleen and Kapha to increase. This effect can allow a Kapha-type dysfunction to be aggravated. Likewise, a Pitta-type aggravation can occur when lying down on the left side, by suppressing Kapha, and allowing Pitta to increase.

Male—Female
Ayurveda classifies a male as being related to positive energy. This includes a connection with Pitta, Fire, Ether and the right side of the body. This is probably the reason why men suffer more from heart attacks (normally a Pitta disorder).

A female is classified as being affected by and related to negative energy. Negative energy (female) is no less important than positive energy (male). Both are essential. As previously explained, the Moon has a strong effect not only on tides but also in the female.

It is interesting to note that recent scientific evidence points to women (especially), being greatly affected when there is a full moon. It has been found that during a full moon, which is a natural phenomenon, police, ambulance and other emergency workers report the greatest number of deaths, injuries and crime. Hospitals too (especially psychiatric ones) have the greatest amount of inmate activity during such time. Psychiatric hospitals have, for a long time, had an unofficial policy of "locking up the place" during a full moon.

The term "lunatic" essentially means a person who is negatively affected by the full moon. This term has been used in society for a very long time.

Science has now "discovered" that through the Moon's influence on the tides and since the human body contains minute seas (70%

water content), the Moon must similarly affect humans. Women (especially Vata types), having a greater amount of negative energy, are therefore greatly affected by lunar energy. The symptoms which can occur are nervousness, stress and temporary mental imbalance (and fluid retention).

Ayurveda has known this for thousands of years, since it is a natural effect and therefore observed in the past. Science is only now confirming things which have been known for thousands of years in India.

Pitta—Kapha

The human body, arbitrarily divided into two parts, is influenced by Pitta and Kapha. In essence, these two forces work together in order to maintain balance in the body. Pitta is akin to hot steam, while Kapha is similar to mud. A major increase in one of these two would then demonstrate a dysfunction akin to its qualities and affect the side of the body related to the humor. For instance, Pitta-type symptoms may be evident on the right side, while Kapha symptoms may show up on the left side.

Pitta is often related to acid conditions (hyperacidity) in the body, while Kapha is akin to alkaline dysfunctions (phlegm, lung congestion).

Essentially then, the two forces working at maintaining a balanced level of health in the body are Pitta and Kapha, the positive and negative factors. Yet, they are both totally lame and ineffective unless controlled by the Vata humor which contains much Prana or life energy.

The Vata humor is the most subtle of the three and consequently attempts to regulate Pitta and Kapha. Vata is the driving force and yet it can also be a cause of dysfunction.

The heat which is a characteristic of Pitta is generally obtained from food which is either hot in temperature or else has an energetically heating effect (like chilies). It is also obtained from the atmosphere and taken into the body via the Surya channel (right nostril) previously described in the text. Likewise, Kapha's coldness is obtained from food and taken into the body via the Ida channel (left nostril).

It is interesting to note also that the female reproductive organ is a Pitta-related energy organ, since it is involved in the menstrual flow of blood (a Pitta tissue). The male reproductive system is Kapha related due to its connection with semen or Kapha seminal fluid. Consequently, although a male is normally Pitta related, his reproductive organs are Kapha related. Likewise, the female is usually under the influence of Kapha, yet her reproductive system is under Pitta.

In this way, a male (Pitta) has an undeniable like-attraction toward's the female's Pitta reproductive organ. A female (Kapha) likewise is attracted to a male's Kapha reproductive organ. If this were not so, Ayurveda explains, there would not be an attraction between male and female.

PART 3

AYURVEDIC PROCESS OF DISEASE

The disease process often follows three paths, akin to the Tridoshas. There is also a strong correlation between the disease process and the Five Elements, and their cycles of interactions, called Wheels.

These three paths are as follows:
1. (Samchaya)—Increase or accumulation of humor (dosha).
2. (Prakopa)—Aggravation of humor.
3. (Prashama)—Alleviation of humor.

Humors continuously rise and fall while undergoing everyday changes. These changes are primarily due to the increase of Prana at a humor-related organ for a set period of time. The second cause is due to increases caused by qualities and substances similar to the humor's qualities. Vata can be increased, for instance, by eating dry fruits. A person of Pitta constitution may increase this humor by eating acidic foods.

Aggravation will indicate an increase in the humor's characteristics to the extent of causing noticeable symptoms, which may result in excess gas or wind for Vata.

Alleviation will signal a point where the person has moved from the aggravated stage back to its former level. This will tend to eliminate the symptoms which had previously appeared.

During the process of digestion, the humors tend to rise and fall as a sine wave, accumulating as follows:

Vata accumulates when food is in the small intestine (Pitta organ), being provoked or aggravated when food is in the large intestine (Vata organ) and alleviated when it is in the stomach (Kapha organ). Consequently, a Vata person should feel fine while ingesting the food, may begin to feel discomfort when food reaches the small intestine, and may definitely feel worse when it finely reaches the large intestine, Vata's source organ.

When food has reached the large intestine of a Pitta person, he/she may feel alleviation of Pitta symptoms, yet may commence to feel unwell when food is in the stomach, and aggravated when it reaches the small intestine, Pitta's source organ.

Food that reaches the small intestine tends to alleviate Kapha. It causes accumulation of Kapha when food is in the large intestine, and is aggravated when it appears in the stomach, Kapha's source organ.

These effects may cause nausea and vomiting for Kapha directly after eating, heartburn two hours later (Pitta) and intestinal gas and distention several hours later (Vata) when food has reached the large intestine.

After the increase or aggravation of the three humors by provoking factors, Agni or the digestive fire weakens, thereby providing an ideal condition for toxins—Ama (undigested food particles) to develop and extend along with the vitiated humor. Ama tends to block the channels and become deposited in weakened areas of the body. This tends to make any treatment more complicated. Ama accumulation with the particular humor is termed Sama (sa= with, ama). No Ama but clearly an unbalanced humor is termed Nirama (Nir= without ama).

HUMOR AFFECTING FACTORS

Vata

Accumulation: Dryness with heat (heat helps to stir Vata) or other Vata promoting qualities.
Aggravation: Coldness.
Alleviation: Heat and wetness (opposite qualities to Vata).

Pitta

Accumulation: Bile qualities (e.g. sharpness, lightness and oiliness).
Aggravation: Heat.
Alleviation: Cold and slowness or dullness (e.g. cold bitters and alterative herbs).

Kapha

Accumulation: Cold and phlegm attributes (e.g. dampness, heaviness and dullness).
Aggravation: Kapha qualities and heat (heat helps to stir Kapha).
Alleviation: heat, dryness, lightness (anti-Kapha).

DISEASE PROCESS

The humors tend to accumulate at their primary organs, that is the:
• Large Intestine for Vata
• Small Intestine for Pitta
• Stomach for Kapha.
Concurrently, three other factors can also occur:
(1) Dislike to qualities which increased them.
(2) Need for substances of opposite characteristics.
(3) Movement out of their primary sites and invasion of various tissues and organs (like a flood).

There will be a dislike of foods or substances similar or like the ones which caused the accumulation.

The natural need or desire for opposite types of substances which will decrease the humor, will be quite pronounced.

Aggravation will then tend to lead towards further complications not only affecting the organ of primary site but also other tissues and organs.

A person of Vata type constitution, when suffering from a Vata dysfunction, will dislike cold and dry-types of foods: e.g. melon, dry fruits. At the same time, the person will be attracted to substances which normally decrease the humor (e.g. musk oil or similar Vata alleviating substances). On continuation of Vata aggravation, the problem will often reach other tissues, like the joints (or other weak points of the body) and will cause dryness of joints and consequent pain in the area (as in arthritis).

The humors must be returned to their site of accumulation for alleviation, and for total eradication of dis-ease. Ayurveda has a thorough method of eradicating the dis-ease by cleaning out the primary sites or the three hollow organs—stomach, small intestine and large intestine. This cleansing procedure is called Pancha Karma, the "Five Therapies". A very careful method of therapeutic vomiting to expel Kapha from the stomach, purgation to eradicate Pitta from the small intestine, and enema treatments to dispel Vata from the colon are usually undertaken. These cleansings follow carefully prepared introductory treatments (massage and sauna type). However, there will be times when Pancha karma will not be suitable and where acupuncture may provide a better alternative. These contra-indications include old age, childhood, debility, heart disease, bleeding, menstruation, ulcerative colitis, organ prolapse, diabetes, acute fevers, enlarged spleen, lymphatic congestion, diarrhea, etc.

Knowledge of the aggravated humor will allow acupuncture treatment of the primary site organ. This means that the stomach can be treated for Kapha, small intestine for Pitta and large intestine for Vata, by puncturing the appropriate organ channel (nadi). This will tend to balance the organ and allow the natural healing forces of the body to expel the accumulated substances.

By balancing the appropriate hollow organ, any toxins which are retained within are allowed to exit. Accumulations of toxins elsewhere in the tissues are no longer restrained there by the pressure held in the hollow organ. The additional use of bitter and pungent herbs can assist in dislodging the toxins (ama) from the tissues, and help to burn them up or expel them. Due to the Wind-Ether elements of bitter herbs, Ama is dislodged and due to the Fire and Wind elements of pungent herbs, it is burned up or consumed as these two also help to rekindle Agni, the digestive fire.

Massage can also assist in channelling Ama (toxins) out of the body by improving circulation.

This is why Acupuncture is an accessory but extremely important therapy.

AGGRAVATION OF HUMORS

Humors are aggravated according to the following priority list:
1. Mental and emotional factors (stress).
2. Diet.
3. Lifestyle.
4. Environmental factors.

Number one on the list has consequence in aggravating the humors the most, while the environmental factors (number 4) normally have the least. In other words, environmental factors take longer to affect the humor than emotional factors. This is why (emotional) stress can be the underlying cause of most diseases. Mental or emotional factors, due to their direct connection with Prana via its subtle qualities, are the most likely to aggravate first.

During the last several years there has been a proliferation of many types of diseases. Most of the patients who attend the clinic suffer primarily from some form of stress. This stress is the emotional factors which we have mentioned above. As stress levels in our society increase, so will the incidence of disease. The stress factors are anger, hate, fear, frustration, anxiousness, etc. In a current report, unemployed youths of a major district of South Australia were found to require more surgical operations than in districts where the unemployment levels were lower. Obviously, the stress caused by unemployment led to the necessity for surgery.

The second most prevalent imbalance-causing factor is diet. Due to the current trend of eating junk foods and adding synthetic chemicals and additives to food, increased prescriptions of synthetic chemical drugs, our diet today is by far the worst ever. Fifty to one hundred years ago, the foods were more organic and pure. Synthetic chemicals were hardly ever used. Irradiation of foods by microwave energy and other similar processes kill the pranic energy which exists in natural foods. This pranic energy therefore becomes deficient in the human body.

The third factor is lifestyle. Due to the two factors previously outlined and the faster pace of our lives today, society is slowly poisoning itself. Our lifestyle has a more hectic pace and can influence our health. The lifestyle includes loud music, eating while watching television or with loud noises, over indulgence in physical exercises where the nervous system can be overtaxed, excessive, prolonged work schedules, no time for reflection or meditation, excessive partying, etc.

The last is environmental factors, which include the weather, living standards and other similar conditions. In some cases, environmental factors nowadays contribute to our ills like never before. Pollution, for instance, allows greater oxidation of foods and tissues. Antioxidants are therefore in vogue today, but are they also synthetic and adding to the problem?

Environmental (atmospheric) factors of a natural kind can be divided into six natural types. When in excess, they can aggravate the appropriate humor (which has a similar quality).

(1) Dryness—Prana
(2) Summer heat—Ether
(3) Wind—Wind
(4) Heat—Fire
(5) Dampness—Water
(6) Cold—Earth

Unfortunately, our society is badly unbalanced in all four contributing factors. Our grandparents may have had only to contend with one or perhaps two of these factors. Today we suffer from all of their effects.

It is therefore imperative that we:

(a) Do not retain built-up emotions or tension, like anger and hate.

(b) Attain a more organic and better diet. Eat foods which are suitable for the constitution and not just because they happen to be natural. Always remember, that fruit/vegetables available out of season may not be as good for us as those only available when in season. There is a reason for nature to have imposed seasonal conditions on some foods.

(c) Take more time out to relax and meditate. Slow down the frantic pace, and perhaps practice more meditative activities like Yoga or Tai Chi. Breathe deeply and slowly as often as possible (intake of Prana).

(d) Ensure to take appropriate action to balance the humors during the various seasons of the year. Pitta should watch out for summer, Kapha for winter and spring, and Vata for autumn. The seasons are a natural means of diagnosis, so that they highlight the internal condition of the body. The appearance of a cold, for instance, is a natural indication that the person has a build-up of toxins and unwanted material which the body needs to expel. Suppressing the cold ensures that these undesirables are retained, and they form the basis of more serious medical problems in the near future. A famous professor once said the seasons are "your own, free medical practitioner."

As a preventive measure, we should indulge in regular massage or acupuncture treatments to balance the system and retain health. It is normally recommended that each person should have a preventive treatment at least once a month.

SIX STAGES OF DISEASE

(1) Accumulation

The causes of accumulation in the respective site are psychological/emotional factors, incorrect diet, lifestyle or environmental effects.

PITTA—Small Intestine. Fever, burning feeling, hyperacidity, yellow urine or feces, irritability and anger, bitter taste. The patient seeks coolness.

VATA—Large intestine. Abdominal distention, constipation, fear, fatigue, dryness, insomnia. The patient seeks warmth.

KAPHA—Stomach. Tiredness, bloating, paleness, heaviness, indigestion. The patient seeks food of a light nature.

(2) Aggravation

Increase of humors in their respective sites increases the strength of symptoms, and reflects symptoms elsewhere in the body.

PITTA—Much acidity and regurgitation, abdominal (burning) pain, great thirst, loss of strength and insomnia.

VATA—Constipation, pain or spasms in abdomen, noises, wind and distention of abdomen.

KAPHA—Lack of appetite, nausea, indigestion, salivation, heavy feeling in the head and chest areas and sleeping to excess.

(3) Flooding

The humors, after filling up their respective sites of accumulation and after being aggravated further, begin to overflow into the rest of the body by a flooding action, especially via the blood. They are still general symptoms not quite localized in one area.

PITTA—Inflamation of skin, headaches (temporal type), conjunctivitis, high fevers, dizziness, vomiting of bile and burning-type diarrhea.

VATA—Dry skin, stiffness and pain in joints, pain in lower back, spasms, headaches (especially in the occipital area and top of the head), convulsions, dry coughs, intermittent-type fevers, abdominal pain and constipation.

KAPHA—Cough, labored breathing, swollen glands, swelling of joints, low grade fevers, mucus in the feces, vomiting.

(4) Displacement

Humors reposition themselves in other sites which are often the most weak and vulnerable in the body. These weaknesses are often

inherited (constitution) and sometimes created by the person him/
herself. The symptoms are of a more specific nature as in (arthritic
type) pain in the joints. The displacement often is to targeted areas
which belong to each individual constitution.

(5) Manifestation

Humors manifest specific symptoms which can be readily recognized as clinical indications or disease names (e.g. arthritis, asthma etc.).
This is the stage that perhaps modern medicine tends to recognize
and then tries to treat. Usually symptoms experienced before this stage
are often delegated by the medical practitioner as "it is all in your head"
or "there is nothing wrong with you." This tends to apply to about
eighty percent of patients visiting medical practitioners. However,
given time, the symptoms will totally manifest and then when it is
obvious, the pronouncement of a disease is then carried out. Isn't this
leaving things a bit too late?

As an example, a male patient attended the clinic wanting to give
up smoking by acupuncture treatment. Diagnosis showed a definite
imbalance in the heart and prognosis was not too good, in our opin-
ion. The patient was requested to seek his medical physician for
further tests. Upon failure of the medical system tests to demonstrate
anything wrong in the heart, the patient was told to go away and
avoid "quacks". He did not return to our clinic ever again.

Approximately eight months later, a new female patient approached
the clinic for treatment. It appeared as though she was a friend of the
first patient who wanted to give up smoking. We were told by her
that the male patient, after being pronounced to have a "healthy"
heart by the medical system, had in fact suddenly died of a heart
attack about six months after his visit to our clinic. The female
patient commented: "Well Doctor, you obviously saw something that
the others didn't see? That's why I am here now!"

(6) Flowering

Unless the underlying factor is healed, the symptoms will diver-
sify or progress to other sites, and the humors will there manifest their

own characteristics. Complex symptoms will then develop as in arthritic pain with degeneration of joints and bones. This can be considered as the chronic stage of disease and one which will take much time and effort to improve, if at all.

It is fitting, that the concept of the six stages of disease outlined above normally resembles the Wheel of Destruction of the Five Elements.

PRANA

(1) Accumulation is analogous to Prana. It is the most subtle commencement of disease since Prana is the most subtle force. The symptoms at this stage are the most mild and least physical (general discomfort).

ETHER

(2) Aggravation is akin to Ether, since this element is more physical than Prana. Aggravation is more physical than accumulation, but still it is subtle. The symptoms are then stronger.

WIND

(3) Flooding is much like Wind, since this element causes movement into other areas. This occurs because the offending humor has completely filled its site of accumulation. Wind helps it to overspill into other parts of the body, although still not localized.

FIRE

(4) Displacement is like Fire. Since this element stirs the unbalanced humor (dosha) which has been taken into other locations by Wind, it then helps to take a hold there.

WATER

(5) Manifestation is analogous to Water, since it is the physical manifestation. Water is the second most physical element. This then forms a disease entity which can be recognized. Water is the element of cohesion, allowing the disease a full foothold.

EARTH
(6) Flowering is similar to Earth, since this is the most physical element and the imbalance has reached its most physical form. The solidification and diversification (Earth) of the imbalance into a full-blown disease with other symptoms has now occurred. Symptoms represented there can now be correlated to qualities of the three humors (doshas) when unbalanced.

WHEEL OF DESTRUCTION	DISEASE STAGES
1. Prana	Accumulation
2. Ether	Aggravation
3. Wind	Flooding
4. Fire	Displacement
5. Water	Manifestation
6. Earth	Flowering

DISEASE PATHWAYS
Ayurveda recognizes three disease pathways.[5] A disease normally enters the first, then leads into the second and finally ends in the third pathway, which is then the deepest form of the disease.

The body's disease pathways mirror the humors as follows:

(1) Inner pathway is connected with Kapha.

(2) Outer pathway is connected with Pitta.

(3) Central pathway is connected with Vata.

Inner Pathway (Kapha)
This consists of the storer or hollow organs of the body, but specifically those dealing with the process of digestion: stomach, small intestine and large intestine—which comprise the gastro-intestinal tract. Through food and water, the humors accumulate, are aggravated and develop in these three. These are superficial types of symptoms and normally are easy to treat. This pathway is the most superficial and in contact with the external world. It relates to Earth and Water, since food normally consists of these two elements and they are first digested before the other elements.

Outer Pathway *(Pitta)*

As an imbalance continues, the next or outer pathway becomes involved and consists of the skin, blood and lymphatics. It is essentially dealing with the circulatory system. At this point we encounter the second most difficult problem to treat. This pathway relates to Fire and Water. Skin rashes, circulation and lymphatic problems normally appear in this Outer pathway.

Central Pathway *(Vata)*

This consists of the inner tissues like bone, muscle etc., as they are found between the inner and outer pathways. This is the last stage of disease and hardest to treat. It usually relates to Vata, as this humor deals with degeneration.

The Central Disease Pathway affects the inner organs and tissues, and is more deep-seated than the other two. Using this logic then, a Vata disease, like degenerative arthritis with wearing away of bones is more difficult to treat than a disease relating to Kapha, like a common cold.

The most complicated and difficult disease to treat is that which involves all three pathways and the three humors, and which has reached the sixth stage of disease. This occurs in cancer.

PROVOCATION DURING TIMES OF DAY

During the day, the humors can be aggravated as follows:

Kapha is provoked during the morning and evening.

Pitta is provoked during midday and midnight.

Vata is provoked during the afternoon and early morning.

Each humor can be alleviated by the period immediately following it, and accumulates during the period before it.

Provocation is usually severely worse during the morning for Kapha due to excess accumulation, during the night for Pitta and early morning for Vata.

Dosha	Aggravated	Alleviated	Accumulates
Kapha	morning	midday	afternoon
	evening	midnight	early morning
Pitta	midday	afternoon	morning
	midnight	early morning	evening
Vata	early morning	morning	midnight
	afternoon	evening	noon

TYPES OF DISEASES

There are three types of diseases, roughly corresponding to Vata, Pitta and Kapha. These three types are progressive so that one follows the next.

A healthy individual has a strong immune system and a balanced nervous system. The immune system has the power to repair and to destroy unwanted foreign bodies. The nervous system (especially the Autonomic Nervous System) is the communication network by which the immune system can properly function. The nervous system must be balanced before health can be achieved. German medical expert (and Ayurvedic physician) Dr. Horst Poehlmann explains that a specific type of antibody is usually created as a response to a particular type of antigen (foreign body). The body knows which one to produce and dispatch to the area according to the specific antigen present. However, when the area is anesthetized, there is no antibody produced as a response, to fight the antigen. This is explained by the fact that the nervous system in the latter case was not functioning in the arm due to the anesthetic (messages were not sent to the brain to initiate an appropriate response).

Impairment or suppression of the nervous system can similarly impair the immune system, and this is why when under a general anesthetic, the patient must be kept in a totally sterile operating theater environment in order to prevent complications due to temporary lowered immunity. These conditions are not totally necessary if the patient receives acupuncture analgesia during an operation, since the immune system is still functioning via an alert nervous system, everywhere else in the body.

Stress, being a type of nervous energy, can directly attack the nervous system (via Vata), which then prevents correct communication and allows immune suppression.

(1) Acute Diseases

These are imbalances in the human organism and the symptoms are natural reactions of the body while trying to heal itself. These are normally self-limiting imbalances which may include diarrhoea, vomiting, sneezing, belching, fever, inflammation, swelling, congestion, redness and pain. The body is then drastically attempting to rid itself of accumulated poisons. The symptoms are therefore purging reactions which are in most cases totally necessary, although not always desired by the patient. As an example, the normal childhood diseases, like chicken pox, measles, mumps, whooping cough etc. are natural purging actions of the body, which are necessary if the child is to build a strong immune system. Consequently, their suppression (by vaccines, etc.) may result in complications at a later stage of life (this is often termed "echo diseases"). For instance, the triple antigen vaccine (DPT) has been implicated in causing SIDS or Cotdeath in infants according to a recent study. Dr. Viera Scheibner, Ph.D., in a paper titled "Association Between Non-Specific Stress Syndrome, DPT Injections and Cot Death" (2nd Immunization Medical Conference, Canberra, Australia 1991) found that following vaccinations, babies' breathing patterns would radically change, and be reduced to 10 percent of their normal amount.

Dr. Scheibner says:

> *"Initially, we did not know about the controversy surrounding vaccination. We merely observed that vaccination was the single greatest cause of stress in small babies and also the single greatest factor preceeding cot death in a large number of cases. We found numerous scientific reports that vaccinated and unvaccinated children contract the relevant infectious disease at approximately the same rate, or that vaccinated children are even more susceptible*

to the infectious disease. Babies may and do die for up to 25 or more days
after vaccination and still as a consequence of the toxic effects of the vaccines."

Ayurveda believes that these childhood diseases occur due to the
need for the child to shed its temporary protective system inherited
from the mother, in order to develop his/her own.

A fever, for instance, warms the body and creates various reactions
which are contradictory to the proliferation of germs, bacteria etc. This
is similar to boiling some water in order to sterilize it. So a fever is
often necessary for health, but due care should be taken in cases of
prolonged high fever, where the body is depleting itself of nutrients.
A common cold (runny nose, expectoration of phlegm, etc.) is often
necessary for expulsion of toxins and waste, accumulated during
specific seasons. Frequent colds normally demonstrate that toxins are
being ineffectively eliminated and the body needs help.

(2) Chronic Diseases

These are serious imbalances which result from the acute disease
not being resolved correctly. This can often occur from the suppression of the acute symptoms. They invariably are self-perpetuating
and treatment is necessary. By suppressing the acute symptoms with
drugs (e.g. anti-biotics for a cold), chronic diseases develop. Examples
of these include asthma, chronic tonsillitis, acne, bronchitis, etc. If not
treated and eliminated, these diseases will graduate in seriousness, con-
tinuing to retain more and more poisons in the body, with the immune system virtually "throwing its hands in the air and giving up."
Suppression of the acute symptoms can easily be done by poisoning
the immune system either on purpose or otherwise by artificial
chemicals including drugs. The immune system cannot then react
which means that its natural symptoms of redness, inflammation,
pain, swelling and restriction in function in order to aid repair are no
longer allowed expression. The inflammation and pain of symptoms
of tonsillitis may be removed by antibiotics, but retention and build-
up of toxins in the body will increase, causing future chronic health
problems.

(3) Chronic Degenerative Diseases

These are often fatal if not checked, and usually cause gradual degeneration of the body. These include cancer, pneumonia, leukemia, aids, alzheimer's disease, etc. Chronic degenerative diseases are usually the result of suppression of acute symptoms via the immune system, which then evolve into chronic diseases and later become degenerative. This is why statistics demonstrate that in Australia today, like most Western countries, one in three people die from cancer. Yet, this disease is virtually unknown in areas where the Western way of life and medicine have little effect, like parts of Tibet and South America.

It is well known that in the case of AIDS, which is a disease characterized by immune deficiency (low Ojas), only those people who originally have a weak immune system seem to die from complications, while those who have a strong immune system either do not suffer or indeed do not contract HIV. The use of illicit drugs tends to weaken the immune system by damaging the nervous system. Thus, drug addicts are greatly at risk. The immune system cannot function correctly without a correctly functioning nervous system.

In order to treat chronic degenerative diseases, the immune system must be sensitized once again, which will take the disease to the chronic stage. Then it will turn back to the acute stage before health can be restored.

Ms. T appeared at our clinic with chronic depression and wanted natural treatment after trying all forms of allopathic therapies including electric shock therapy, without avail.

After initial treatment and a healthier diet, she began to lose unwanted weight. Also, the depression disappeared as well as several other symptoms. The strange thing was that she suddenly contracted an acute case of tonsillitis and straight away sought medical advice. Antibiotics were prescribed for her condition. The tonsillitis symptoms subsided but the depression returned. After further treatment in our clinic by which the poisons (including antibiotics) were allowed to exit the body, the depression once again totally disappeared and health improved once again. The tonsillitis occurred because the body was once again reacting correctly and was trying to resolve years of accumulated problems. The healing reactions are sometimes referred to as the "healing crisis."

Mrs. C. tried all types of medicines in order to fix her cracking, bleeding skin problem on her hands before turning up at our clinic's doorstep. After treatment, her skin condition improved but she then developed a mild case of diarrhoea. Lucky for her, she did not seek suppressive medication for the diarrhea, which subsided on its own. Immediately after, the skin condition totally improved since the toxins had been allowed a way out of the body (via the diarrhea).

In both cases, the symptoms of diarrhea and tonsillitis were natural symptoms by which the body was trying to rid itself of poisons. Suppression of the symptoms in the first case with antibiotics returned the patient back to her original condition of depression. Non-suppression of the symptoms in the latter case permitted the poisons to exit the body (via diarrhea), and allowed the immune system to heal the original complaint. Needless to say, both patients were more than pleased with the final results.

Ayurveda considers Ojas as the subtle essence of the immune system and as such, when Ojas is low, the immune system is weak. It then allows chronic and degenerative diseases to develop. By increasing Ojas, we produce a strong immune system, and can then remove all traces of chronic or degenerative diseases (in cases where the degeneration can be repaired by the body itself). We must remember though, that while doing so we may experience some natural symptoms, the natural signs of healing.

Ayurveda believes that not only wrong diets, lifestyle etc. can interfere with the health process, causing a dysfunction, but that external factors like contagious epidemics can sometimes similarly affect the person. In most cases though, Ayurveda believes that these epidemics will generally affect those with a lowered immune system, especially children, infirmed and old people. Epidemics usually never kill all the population of an affected region, but instead only those most at risk. When the West first entered into Japan, the healthy population did not become affected by Western diseases, but only those people who were more at risk. Ayurveda also believes that a bad seed (disease) can only grow in soil which allows it to grow (unhealthy body). By increasing immunity and balancing the nervous system, most, if not all, of these dysfunctions can be prevented or eliminated.

Notes:

1. *Charaka Samhitta,* XXVI [10].
2. *Ibid.,* p. 452)
3. *Ibid.,* p. 452)
4. *Ibid.,* Vol. 1, p. 463.

CHAPTER VI

DIAGNOSIS

In Ayurvedic medicine, there are many and varied forms of diagnostic procedures. The whole body continues to output information about the internal conditions by various means and in many areas of the body. Observation and proper deduction of these signs allowed the ancient ayurvedic physicians to formulate their forms of diagnosis.

The body has an internal language which has to be correctly interpreted to be understood. The physician is in fact an interpreter who reads the signs and translates them into human language. These signs include pain, inflammation, fever and physical marks which appear or affect various parts of the body. These areas relate to organs, humors, etc. so that their location can be useful in diagnosing the area affected. For instance, pain in the back of the leg (sciatica) can often demonstrate an imbalance of Vata, affecting the Bladder channel and the kidney.

As a result, Ayurveda outlines three procedures for diagnosis. Every form of diagnosis slots into one of these three. These are generally carried out during every Ayurvedic diagnostic consultation.

1. Observation *(Darshana)*
Any procedure which involves observing an area of the body, whether it be the eye/iris, ear, tongue, face, etc. in order to ascertain the exact cause of disease is referred to as observation.

2. Palpation *(Sparshana)*
Palpation involves probing, touching or tapping the body, and includes procedures such as pulse reading, auricular, body and abdominal marma point palpation.

3. Questioning *(Prashna)*
Questioning (also called interrogation) involves finding out infor-

mation about the patient, either from the patient him/herself or else an attendant. Family history may often be necessary in order to ascertain a common hereditary thread for the disease or complaint in question.

COMMON DIAGNOSES

1. Tongue observation.
2. Pulse palpation.
3. Iris and eye observation.
4. Facial signs.
5. Abdominal palpation.
6. Body marma points palpation.
7. Ear points (auricular) palpation.
8. Urine and saliva analysis.
9. Lips observation.
10. Finger/toe nails observation.

Palpation of the whole abdominal area can identify areas of pain, inflammation etc. according to the anatomical position of the underlying organs like the liver, intestines and spleen. Coldness would relate to congestion and lack of flow of blood, primarily caused by a lack of flow of Prana through the channels.

Palpation of the major lymph nodes can similarly identify congestion in the lymphatic system when pain sensitivity is present there.

Referred pain is the pain which is located in an area remote to the source of the problem. For instance, science knows that a liver dysfunction can demonstrate pain in the right shoulder, between the neck and arm. Lung dysfunction can show pain on the left side of the shoulders, opposite to the liver. The body, via the channels, has other referred types of pain and symptoms which, when understood, can demonstrate the source of the problem, normally remote from the location of the symptom.

Correct massage of the lymph nodes in the breast area, especially in women, can often serve as a preventive measure against lumps and tumors. Breast examination (including breast self examination, B.S.E.) is important to diagnose the existence of lumps etc, but lymphatic massage of the breasts will often prevent lumps from developing in the first place.

A complete and thorough examination is therefore required to be carried out with every new patient. The diagnostic procedures outlined above can therefore assist in attaining a true picture of the patient and his/her malady.

PULSE DIAGNOSIS *(Nadi Pariksha)*

In order to ascertain the internal imbalances of the body, Ayurveda recommends various diagnostic procedures. One of these is the Pulse Diagnosis (Nadi Pariksha) which is often taken at the site of the radial bone/artery in the arm (Fig. 14). It should be explained that since the pulses deal with minute amounts of energetic currents which, like electricity, are invisible, their detection requires experience and practice. An experienced safecracker develops a similar sensitivity by constant practice over a long time, in order to open combination safes.

The radial pulse at the wrist site contains three positions which highlight the conditions of the three humors: Vata, Pitta and Kapha. An imbalance in one of these humors will demonstrate a certain quality in the pulse, at the appropriate location.

The word Nadi which normally means channel or conduit is also translated as "pulse" because it is via the nadis (pranic channels) that the radial pulses receive information about the internal condition of the humors or indeed the organs.

The humors are located in both wrists according to their physical positioning in the body. Vata is found at the first point of both wrists, which represents the lowest area of the trunk, the Vata Area. This is the area below the navel which relates to Vata and its related organs like the kidney, large intestine and reproductive system.

Pitta is found in the middle position of the wrist and is found in the middle position of the trunk. This is the area between the navel and the breathing diaphragm.

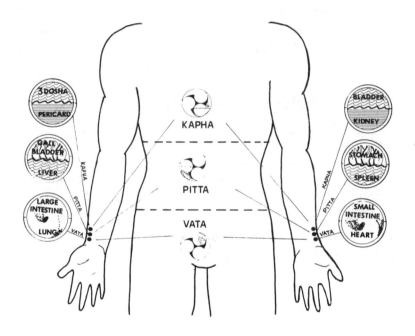

Fig. 14 The Organ and Humor Pulses

Kapha is located at the last or third point in a similar manner to the trunk. This is the area above the breathing diaphragm, or highest portion of the human trunk.

QUALITIES

The humoral pulses have unique qualities which allow a practitioner to correctly identify them.

Vata

When Vata is aggravated, the quality of the pulse has a snake-like, slithering feel. This tends to be erratic, with mostly uneven pulses, including missed heartbeats. Vata aggravation usually leads to a very fast heartbeat, somewhere above 80 beats per minute. The more Vata is unbalanced the more Vata-type the pulse becomes. In fact, at the time of death which is the Vata stage, the pulse can reach 160 beats per minute. Vata has an irregular, feeble, fast pulse.

Pitta

When Pitta is aggravated, the feel of the pulse has a definite frog-like movement. This is similar to the feeling of jumping on a "Pogo stick"—that is: "poing, poing, poing, poing." It is prominent and mostly even. The aggravation of Pitta demonstrates a heartbeat of 70-80 beats per minute. Pitta has a prominent, jumping, excited pulse, which not only resembles a jumping frog but also the flaring of a fire (with which it is related).

Kapha

When Kapha is aggravated, it demonstrates the graceful movements of a swan. It is generally soft and even. When aggravation of Kapha occurs, the heartbeat tends to also be affected; it is usually under 65 beats per minute. Consequently, Kapha aggravation leads to extreme relaxation; no "get-up and go." Kapha has a slow, strong and regular pulse and often resembles the movement of a river (Water) with which it is related.

PULSE QUALITIES IN SUMMARY

Superficial pulse: The pulse response when superficial pressure is applied. Loss of pulse detection occurs when deep pressure is applied. This type of pulse is usually indicative of acute conditions of an external nature.

Deep pulse: Pulse responds to deep pressure but is not obvious at a superficial level. This occurs with dysfunctions of a deep seated nature, affecting the interior organs and systems—the Central Disease Pathway.

Fast pulse: Indicative of Vata or Pitta syndromes. Vata will be fast and weak, while Pitta will be fast and strong. Excessive rapid pulse is nevertheless related to Vata syndromes.

Slow pulse: Indicative of a Kapha syndrome. Generally, it is 60 bpm or less with a broad and even nature.

Medium pulse: A pulse between 60-80 bpm is indicative of Pitta syndromes. This pulse is strong like a jumping frog.

Irregular pulse: An irregular or missed beat pulse is indicative of Vata syndromes, that is, with the quality of the Wind.

Wiry pulse: A wiry pulse feels as though you are pressing on a tight guitar string. It is taut and forceful. Normally this occurs with Fire syndromes.

Rolling pulse: A rolling pulse is the Kapha type pulse which is smooth, flowing and forceful.

Thready pulse: This is the fine pulse of Vata.

TAKING THE PULSE

When taking the pulse, the physician will place the first, middle and ring fingers on the three locations of the radial pulse of the patient, just below the radial (wrist) bone. The patient's wrist should be relaxed and slightly flexed. The first finger of the physician on the first position, will detect Vata because according to Ayurveda this finger represents and is related to the Wind element. The middle finger, being connected to the Fire element is best able to detect Pitta at the middle position. The ring finger on the third position detects Kapha because it is related to the Water element. In reality, each of the five digits is related to one of the Five Elements and their order of appearance is according to the Wheel of Creation (Fig. 15). The thumb relates to the first element Ether, the index to Wind, the middle finger to Fire, ring finger to Water and lastly, the little finger to Earth, the last most physical element.

The more unbalanced or aggravated the humor, the more prominent will be the pulse at the appropriate location. This tends to be more noticeable at the first location (index finger) or Vata point for Vata, the second point (middle finger) for Pitta, and the third point (ring finger) for Kapha. Besides the location of the prominent pulse, the quality of the pulse should also be taken into account, which together will normally occur.

Traditionally, the pulse of a male is taken on the right wrist because Ayurveda outlines the right side of the body as the Pitta, male side. The female is taken on the left wrist, as this is the (Kapha) negative, female side. It is often that male patients will tend to have more prominent pulses on the right wrist, while females will appear on the left. However, the pulses should be taken on both sides of the body, that is, the right and left radial pulses for each patient. Normally three readings are taken when examining the pulse. The pressure of the three fingers must be even to insure a correct reading.

Organ Pulses

Not only does the radial pulse reflect the balance or imbalance of the three humors, they also demonstrate the conditions of each of the major human organs. This is achieved by the pulses' connection with the organs via a set of internal pranic channels which connect with the pulse and carry pranic currents:

> *"These currents circulate through the blood, passing through the vital organs such as the liver, kidney, heart. By feeling the superficial and deep pulsations, the sensitive examiner can detect the conditions of these various organs."*[1]

The deep pressure on the radial pulse always detects the condition of the solid organs—for example, the liver, heart and kidney. Super-

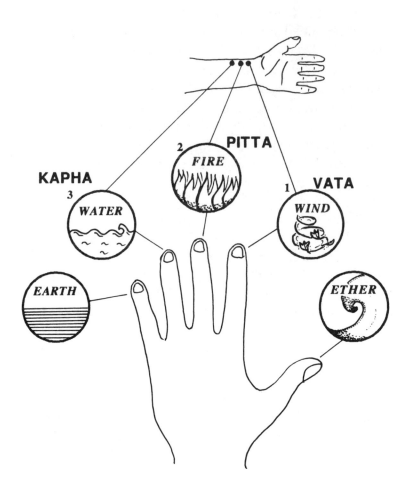

Fig. 15 The Pulses and the Five Elements

ficial pressure detects the hollow organs—e.g. the small and large intestines, bladder and stomach.

The location of each organ on the radial pulse is according to, and dependent on, the Five Elements and the physical location of each solid organ in the body. Where the organ, such as the heart, is located in the chest (thoracic) area, the organ is detected in the first pulse location. If the organ is in the middle position of the trunk, it is similarly located in the middle position of the three pulses. Where the organ, such as the kidney, is located below the navel, then it is located on the third position of the pulse.

First pulse location

The heart located in the thoracic cavity is positioned in the first location of left wrist.

As the lung is physically located also in the thoracic area, it is found in the first position of the right wrist.

Second pulse location

The liver is in the middle position, on the *right* side of the trunk. It is found in the middle position of the *right* wrist.

Likewise, the spleen is located in this middle position but on the *left* side of the trunk. It is located in the middle position of the *left* wrist.

Third pulse location

The kidney is physically located in the lower aspect of the trunk so that it is found in the third pulse position of the left wrist.

Some ancient experts also attribute the third position of the right wrist pulse to the kidney (since there are two of these organs in the body). Some other experts relate the third position of the right wrist pulses to the pericardium, an organ which is energetically related to Kapha (Water) or fluid flow in the body. The pericardium is also connected with the heart, since it is the sack which surrounds the latter.

The other type of organs (the hollow ones), are located in the pulses according to their connection with the Five Elements. Where an organ is related to a particular element, it is found in the same location as its related solid organ. For instance, since the small intestine is related to the heart due to the Fire element, these two organs are located in the same pulse location (first position, left wrist). This also applies to the other organs. The solid organs are detected with deep pressure, while the hollow organs are detected with superficial pressure.

LEFT Pulse	Superficial	Deep	Related Element
1.	Small Intestine	Heart	Fire
2.	Stomach	Spleen	Earth
3.	Bladder	Kidney	Water (Vata)

RIGHT Pulse	Superficial	Deep	Related Element
1.	Large Intestine	Lung	Wind
2.	Gallbladder	Liver	Ether
3.	Tridosha	Pericardium	Water

TONGUE DIAGNOSIS (Jihva)

The tongue, like other parts of the body, can be utilized in our quest for a correct diagnosis. The state of health of the body is continuously reflected on the tongue, as it is on the pulses, and much information can be gathered from it. This information includes the condition of the gastro-intestinal tract, unbalanced humors and organs and accumulation of toxins (undigested particles of digestion: Ama). Also, information on nutritional deficiencies and emotional imbalances can be found.

Tongue proper: The tongue itself can reveal information on the three humors (Fig. 16). It resembles the constitutional attributes such as a thin, small/long trembling tongue for Vata, a large, thick and roundish tongue for Kapha and a medium sized tongue for Pitta. Markings on the tongue can be correlated with dysfunctions in the major organs and or parts of the body.

Color: The color of the tongue, normally pink in health also reveals similar information.

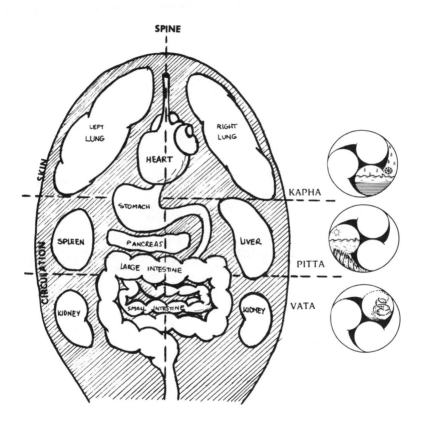

Fig. 16 The Tongue—Organ and Humor Locations

Vata shows a pale tongue (normal lack of heat for Vata).

Pitta demonstrates a reddish tongue (heat).

Kapha shows a pale and whitish tongue (lack of heat).

Coating

The coating on the tongue (usually very thin or nonexistent in a healthy body) shows possible accumulation of toxins along with possible aggravation of the humors. A thick tongue coating indicates a mass build-up of toxins in the body.

Thick/white coating—represents accumulation of toxins (Ama).

Yellow/greasy coating—shows Ama fermentation with possible heat build up. Possible sodium phosphate deficiency.

Brown/black coating—Vata aggravation.

Yellow coating—Pitta aggravation (with some Ama).

White/mucous coating—Kapha aggravation and possible potassium chloride deficiency.

Vata dysfunctions may lead to dry tongue due to this humor's characteristic. Cracks on the tongue are usually attributed to chronic derangement of Vata or excess high Pitta (heat).

Pitta imbalances may lead to a red and dry tongue due to heat energy consuming fluids. In a condition which includes toxins (Ama), the tongue will be moist.

Kapha imbalances are usually indicated by excessive mucous or moisture on the tongue.

Geography of humors

The tongue can be divided into three sections in accordance with the three humors. It also mirrors the way these are located in the trunk. Kapha is located above the diaphragm (in the thorax), as well as in the area near the tip of the tongue (which correlates with the thoracic area).

The area of Pitta ranges from the breathing diaphragm to the navel in the trunk. This is mirrored in the area of the middle of the tongue.

Vata is located near the back of the tongue which represents the lower area of the trunk, below the navel.

Geography of organs

The tongue not only reflects the humors in their appropriate locations, but it also reflects the human organs. These are located according to their positions in the human trunk, with the tip of the tongue being the area below the neck and the back of the tongue representing the lower part of the trunk. For example, the heart is reflected near the tip, the liver on the middle position right side, and the kidneys in the area at the back of the tongue. Imbalances and diseases normally show various symptoms on the tongue which can assist diagnosis.

The spleen is found on the left side of the middle of the tongue, directly across from the liver which is positioned on the right side.

The small intestine is found in the middle area at the back of the tongue, in much the same manner found in the trunk. The large intestine is positioned like its trunk counterpart, ascending on the right side, transversing across and descending on the left side of the tongue.

The lungs are also located near the tip of the tongue on either side of the heart.

Where a discoloration or sign is found on a particular part of the tongue, then this organ is afflicted by an imbalance, according to the characteristics demonstrated. For instance, much redness in the heart area of the tongue may indicate excessive heat in the heart (excess Pitta). Depressions in the lung area of the tongue may indicate delicate lungs. Toxins in the large intestine may show up as a white coating on the appropriate area of the tongue.

The spinal column is found in the middle of the tongue, from the tip to the back of the tongue. When an imbalance occurs in the spine or when emotions are retained which affect this area, signs will appear here. For instance, if a deviation occurs in the middle line (of the tongue) then the appropriate area in the spine is affected.

A patient attended the clinic. Upon looking at the tongue during diagnosis, the line along the middle of the tongue was found to kink at least in three positions. This relates to three problems in the spine. The patient was referred for chiropractic treatment. Without a word being mentioned, the chiropractor explained to the patient that she had three problems in the spine, the same number and locations that we had located. Through our own individual methods, we both arrived at the same diagnostic conclusion.

Observation of the tongue proper, the coating and geographic position of any imbalance, will demonstrate a correct diagnosis. In combination with other forms (like the pulses), the tongue can form a powerful tool of differential diagnosis.

The tongue reflects the internal conditions of the organs, humors and systems, and is believed to be connected with them via a network of pranic channels (nadis).

Recently, various investigators have found that puncturing the tongue at strategic locations, according to the plan outlined above, does indeed achieve a therapeutic effect on the afflicted organ. Heart problems were cured by needling the area of the heart on the tongue, etc. However, there is some doubt in the West about regular treatment directly on the tongue, as most patients would find it most uncomfortable holding the tongue outside of the mouth for any length of time while receiving acupuncture treatment.

EAR DIAGNOSIS (Karna)

The ear or auricle is a site of Ayurvedic therapy and diagnosis. Fascination with the ear stems back thousands of years, having been recorded three thousand years ago in the Suchi Veda, or "science of acupuncture" text. Contrary to the tongue, the ear is readily accessible to diagnosis and treatment via massaging or needling. Various tender spots can be found in the area according to the organs which are unbalanced. These spots are connected via nadi channels to the appropriate organs (Fig. 17). An imbalance in an organ reflects distention or blood congestion in the ear. A problem in the leg, for instance, can be diagnosed by pressing the (leg) area of the ear with a fine, blunt instrument. This may show slight pain or sensitivity. A needle in this area may release some blood when the needle is removed, demonstrating congestion in the related organ and the ear.

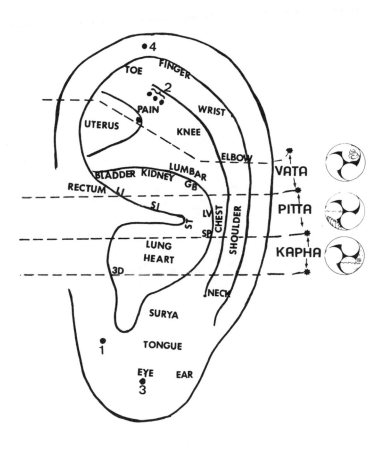

Fig. 17 Some Auricular Marmas

Although the concept of auricular acupuncture in India is ancient, many investigators throughout the years have continued to add knowledge to this system to arrive at what we know today. This is also true of Ayurveda, in general, since it is a science which is alive and without end. Some credit is given today to French neurologist and acupuncturist, Professor Nogier, who first coined the idea that the ear represents an upside-down foetus. Consequently, the points for the organs and limbs in the ear exist according to their image in the body.

One of the modern innovations is to name marmas or acupuncture spots in the ear according to medical terminology of diseases—e.g. asthma spot, lumbago point, sciatica point, etc. These names were not originally utilized by Ayurvedic physicians of the past, but of course should be incorporated in any auricular acupuncture system today.

Ayurveda explains that the three humors (Vata, Pitta and Kapha) are reflected in the ear according to a similar scheme as outlined in the tongue or pulses.

Vata is positioned in the Vata area of the ear, which (because it represents an upside down foetus) is located in the highest area of the ear (furthermost from the lobe).

The middle position of the ear roughly corresponds with Pitta, while the lower one, just directly above the lobe, corresponds with Kapha. The lobe itself represents the head area of the body.

The organs and other body parts are positioned in much the same manner. The large intestine and kidney are found in the Vata area, the liver and gall bladder in the Pitta area and the lung and heart in the Kapha area of the ear.

There are also other areas of therapeutic value, such as the Pain spot (related to Vata) which treats pain and Vata type nervous disorders. This spot also treats inflammation by cooling down the area. The Surya (Sun) spot can be needled for the treatment of Pitta migraines (temporal headaches). The Tridosha (3D) spot is utilized for treating imbalances of the three humors' mutual harmony. Bronchial asthma is treated at a point on the lobe (1), while hemorrhoids can be helped by treating points in the Vata area (2) next to the Pain spot. The Immune (Ojas) spot (3) near the center of the lobe is normally used to provide increased immunity, especially during childhood and may even increase longevity. Allergies and skin problems can be treated by a point (4) on the helix (top of ear). (Refer to Fig. 17)

Anatomical areas like the arm, leg, chest, neck, eyes, etc. are found in the ear almost in the same manner as they are located in the body.

The needle punctures the ear to a short depth. It does not penetrate through to the other side. The pranic energy circulating through the ear in the channels then takes charge and retains the metal needles in position almost as though it (energy) was a magnet. When the needle falls out from its position, this usually indicates that there is excess negative energy in that organ and so the expulsion of this energy is done by removing the needle. Once the energy has balanced sufficiently, the needle will be retained in the ear for an appropriate length of time. Once it has provided sufficient therapy to the body, the needle in most cases will fall out, or can be easily pulled out without any resistance. If the body has not quite finished, the practitioner will often find the removal of the needle most difficult.

The needles are retained in the ear for approximately 30-60 minutes. Treatment is carried out according to Ayurvedic diagnosis. Thus with a Vata type problem, the Vata organs and related points can be used for therapy. Also, the concept of the Wheel of Support of the Five Elements can similarly be utilized in cases of excess/deficiency syndromes.

Many imbalances and diseases have been successfully treated by ear acupuncture. It is easily performed and the area is normally accessible. This, in combination with needling of the body itself, provides a great source, not only of treatment, but diagnosis also.

Notes:

1. *Ayurveda, The Science of Self-Healing, p. 56.*

CHAPTER VII

PART I
THE ACUPUNCTURE NEEDLE (SUCHI)

Traditionally, many different types of needles were used for acupuncture and surgery. Some were curved, but most were straight. Some were made of gold and some of silver.

The term for needle is "suchi" which evolves from the word "suc" (pronounced sooch) and means "to point out, indicate." As needles were also used for surgery, there were many different types used in India, such as Ara, Kuthari, Atimukha and Badisha. Different lengths and thicknesses were used dependent on the area to be needled.

The original needle was probably not much different from the ones used today for suturing, (long, thin, tubular length of metal or bone). Jurgen Thorwald relates that Ayurveda used bone or bronze needles, both straight and bent.[1] Whereas the suturing needles may have required a small hole for the insertion of a thread and a small curvature along its length for ease in suturing, the needle which was utilized for acupuncture did not require them. Consequently, various versions of acupuncture needles were created over years of practice.

The model of traditional needle which was handed down to the author is in fact a long, thin, tubular needle, with various additions which provide easier handling and multiple features (Fig. 18).

These needles, originally made of gold or silver could not be discarded due to their value, so consequently, they were designed to last, be sterilized and provide multi-functions.

Handle
A needle made out of a long piece of metal (as for suturing) is not comfortable or functional for acupuncture; therefore an appropriate handle is often added. This handle is thicker (in diameter) than the needle and is often (although not always) knurled or patterned to provide a non-slip grip for the fingers. The knurled handle needle

allows scraping with the fingernail in order to promote pranic flow.

Fingerguard

Between the blade of the needle and the handle is often found a fingerguard, which is no more than a spherical metal ball which prevents the fingers from sliding off the handle and onto the blade. Also, it provides a safe stop when fully inserting the needle's blade through the skin, due to its rounded features. The fingerguard represents the chakra—the wheel of nature—and due to its curved surface is safer than a straight edge.

Blade

The blade is a long, tubular, thin strip of metal with a sharp point. This needle point is different from a hypodermic needle in that the suchi is similar to the point of a bullet (rounded) while the hypodermic has a very sharp, angular point. The suchi tends to push aside muscle fibers, etc. when penetrating, while the hypodermic tends to cut through them instead, causing trauma and discomfort.

End

Many needles did not have an end to them, but rather the end was provided by the handle. Others had a spherical type of ball (similar to the finger guard) added to the end of the handle. This provided a stop for the fingers when removing needles. A fascinating addition to the suchi was a spike made out of the same metal which allowed herbs to be spiked on the end of the handle, then lit so that the heat could penetrate into the body of the patient, with the needle as the conductor. The use of burning incense is generally attributed to the allied art of Indian moxibustion (agni-karma) where herbs with aroma were used according to their effects on the three constitutions or humors. The same herbs made into a ball, could be spiked on the needle to add heat. In most cases, a common standard needle with all the above features was desirable and mostly found in practice.

Although in the past, needles were sterilized before re-use, today more and more people are demanding disposable needles. Obvious-

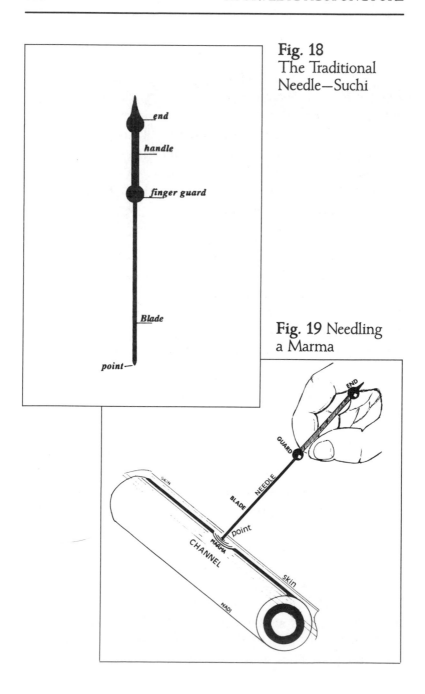

Fig. 18
The Traditional
Needle—Suchi

end

handle

finger guard

Blade

point

Fig. 19 Needling
a Marma

ly the latter ones cannot be made of gold or silver. In order to produce an inexpensive disposable needle, stainless steel is usually prefer-
red. It must be strong, lightweight and flexible.

It is hoped that in the near future, needle manufacturers may also
produce disposable Indian needles. This may also offer an additional
source of income for Indian manufacturers. Currently, Ayurvedic
acupuncturists in the West (and India) must, by necessity, use Japanese
or Chinese-made and designed disposable needles.

Needle Insertion

The needle is inserted to a certain depth with the aid of small rota-
tions, created by the index finger and thumb of the needling hand.
As the needle is rotated it is also pushed in further into the skin (Fig. 19).

While one hand (needling hand) is used to insert the needle, the other
hand assists by either gathering the skin or by steadying the sur-
rounding area. Angle of insertion depends on the area being punctured and effect desired. Needling the area near the face (where bone
is directly beneath the skin) involves a small angle between the
needle and the skin in order to avoid the bone. In areas where there
is more muscle, the needle may penetrate deeper. In the thigh, for instance, the angle of the needle can be at 90 degrees to the skin and
may have deeper penetration due to more muscle availability.

By puncturing against the direction of the channel's energy (Prana)
flow, the amount of energy in the organ or channel can be reduced
if desired. This normally equates with sedating.

By puncturing with the direction of the flow of energy in the channel, the energy will tend to be increased in the channel or organ. This
results in a tonifying effect. These effects are often necessary in excess and deficiency syndromes.

After insertion of the needle in the corresponding marma or point,
the pranic energy will tend to grab the needle point and begin a
therapeutic effect. When Prana "grabs", the needle will become
erect and firm. When this occurs, the needle will not be able to be
removed. After the induction period (up to thirty minutes), the

therapeutic effect will commence. This may continue for up to another thirty minutes, before subsiding. Removal of the needle after only a few minutes of insertion will simply disperse energy, an effect which sometimes may be desired.

Needle polarities

The use of a gold needle was standard in ancient India as it encouraged energy flow due to the heating properties of gold. Just like boiling water has continuous movement due to the heat from the stove, so too gold increases movement by heating. Gold has traditionally been considered as having a positive (heat) effect while silver has a negative (cool) effect.

Ayurveda teaches that these metals have effects on the three humors and their use has to be carefully regulated. Therefore, the type of needle used, whether gold or silver, should be considered in the light of their balancing or unbalancing actions on the humors.

A Pitta person with a major Pitta imbalance may indeed feel worse when gold needles are used. The correct metal for Pitta is therefore silver.

A Kapha person with Kapha imbalances may indeed become worse if silver needles are used. The correct metal for Kapha is gold (heating).

A Vata patient may be assisted by the use of gold needles, since the heating effect will be welcome by Vata's coolness. Likewise, the use of silver needles may similarly help as this metal's calming energy will relax the "nerves" of Vata. However, excess use of either one may aggravate Vata, so caution should be exercised. The use of gold or silver earrings can often have a similar effect.

Depth and Angle of Insertion

Depending on the area which needs to be punctured, the needle may have to be inserted either deeper or more superficially. In areas where there is sufficient muscle mass (thighs, biceps) it can be inserted deeper according to the marma point. This maximum depth is outlined for each marma in Appendix A, at the end of this book.

Traditionally, the fingerguard acted as a stop for the needle. An area where a depth of one inch penetration was required could see a practitioner using a needle with a one-inch long blade and insert it to the full length of the blade, to the fingerguard. As the guard is spherical, it caused no trauma to the skin and was used as a stop guide.

The needles used today are straight, have a long blade and a handle. The blade is normally about 0.30 mm. thick and usually 30 mm long. Other lengths and thicknesses are available. Some people call this type of needle "filiform" (L. filum = thread).

Needles are sometimes inserted at an angle to the skin, in the direction of the flow of Prana in the channel, to increase energy; against the flow to decrease it; and at various angles according to the anatomy of the area of the body. P is for perpendicular to the skin, H is for horizontal and O is for oblique. These are also outlined in Appendix A.

In traditional acupuncture no other device except for a needle or agni stick (moxibustion) was used. Today, practitioners can connect current source devices to artificially mimic the energy flow by providing a fluctuating electric current from a battery source. Each of the two cable leads from the device is connected to one needle to provide a current loop through the body. This device may be used to provide acupuncture analgesia or pain relief. It is also used as a form of anesthetic during various surgical operations.

Laser acupuncture is also in fashion today where a laser light is positioned on the skin at a marma point to stimulate the flow of energy.

PART 2
CHANNELS (NADIS)
NADIS/BIO-ENERGY CHANNELS

"The Shiva Samhita mentions 350,000 nadis [or channels in the human body], of which fourteen are stated to be important."[2]

The fourteen important channels mentioned above are, in fact, the twelve organ channels described earlier in the text and also the two channels called the Governor or Minister (Amatya Nadi) and the Conception (Janma Nadi) channels.

In Ayurvedic acupuncture fourteen major channels (nadis) are considered most important. These are major nadis distributed over the entire human body, which allow Prana to flow. These channels, having great therapeutic value (like the chakras) are found close to the skin, connecting with a major organ internally and externally with tissues, etc., where marmas or pressure points are located. These marmas have low resistance.

By massaging, needling or heating the marmas (strategic vital points), a therapeutic effect can be achieved not only in the local area but also in the organs which are related to these channels.

The nadis are subtle channels which are believed to be made up of three sheaths or layers, and they carry Prana in one form or another as it moves around the body. The nadis are also vehicles for the three humors, Vata, Pitta and Kapha. When a channel's energy flow is impaired, this can cause a similar blockage in the flow of the body fluids like blood, lymph, etc.

The channels delineated as carrying Prana cannot normally be seen, since they carry invisible energy, much like electricity. It is possible that scientific equipment may one day be designed to not only detect but show these channels. Perhaps a whole system of diagnosis can be produced by scanning the various pranic channels without even touching the person, and then utilizing the information to arrive at a computer-based diagnosis and treatment.

Many times, patients complain of pain along a particular limb according to a specific complaint. These areas of pain in most cases can be identified with the pranic channels and trace the same areas that the channels trace. For instance, with heart disease, the area of the Heart channel in the arm is often affected (e.g. during heart attack). With sciatica (a Vata imbalance), the Bladder channel (Vata related) is usually involved. With Pitta type arthritis, the Gallbladder channel (Pitta related) area is involved. With Kapha arthritis, often the Tridosha channel is related (Fig. 20).

The fourteen important channels mentioned above are in fact the twelve organ channels described earlier in the text and also the two channels called the Governor and Conception channels. These two do not relate to a specific organ but have a related effect on an area. The Conception channel for instance controls, is affected by and affects conception—childbirth and the reproductive system. This channel often reflects discomfort (or sensitivity) along its full length in the female during pregnancy.

The twelve major organ channels can be divided into two types: those which are related to the solid organs (like the heart) and those which are related to the hollow organs (like the large intestine). Anatomically, the solid organ channels are always located along the inside of the limbs, while the hollow organ channels are located along the outside or external aspect of the limbs. Consequently, the solid organ channels are referred to as inside channels (Antar Nadis), while the hollow organ channels are called outside channels (Bahya Nadis).

INSIDE CHANNELS—Arm (Antar Nadis)

The inside channels in the arm have their pranic energy flow from the organ to the end of the fingers. The flow of Prana is therefore down along the inside of the arm. These consist of the following organ channels (Fig. 21):

Heart Channel (H)

The Heart channel runs along the inside of the arm, from the heart, along the shoulder and palm to connect with the little finger. There are nine (9) pressure points (marmas) along this channel which can be needled for therapy. The energy flow is from the organ to the finger, so that the first point (marma) is near the heart, the ninth one is in

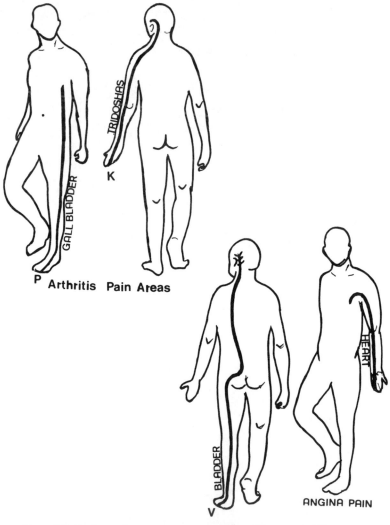

Fig. 20 Referred pain areas and the Channels/Humors

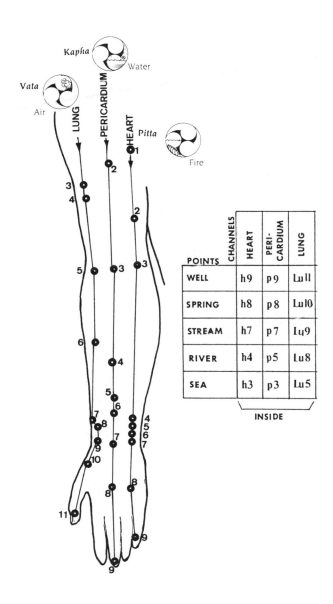

Fig. 21 The Inside Arm Channels (and their vital points)

the tip of the little finger. The Heart channel is needled for heart, Pitta and some mental disorders (the heart affects the mind).

Pericardium Channel (P)

The Pericardium channel runs parallel to the Heart channel, but along the middle of the inside of the arm. Like the Heart channel, its energy flow is from the pericardium to the end of the middle finger. There are nine (9) pressure points (marmas) also along this channel which are used for therapy. The first point starts near the nipple, on the chest while the ninth is at the tip of the middle finger.

Lung Channel (L)

The Lung channel also runs parallel to the Heart and the Pericardium channels but this time along the thumb area of the arm. Being an inside channel of the arm, the energy flow occurs from the lung to the thumb. There are eleven (11) pressure points (marmas) along its length which can be used for therapy. The first point occurs on the upper chest area, while the eleventh point is located at the side of the thumb (near the nail).

OUTSIDE CHANNELS—Arm *(Bahya Nadis)*

The outside channels which occur along the arm are found along the back of the hand. The three outside channels of the arm refer to the hollow organs: small intestine (Pitta), tridosha (Kapha) and large intestine (Vata) (Fig. 22).

The channels' energy flow direction is opposite to the inside channels so, consequently, it commences near the fingers in the channels and travels in an upward arm direction.

Small Intestine (S.I.)

The Small Intestine channel is directly behind the Heart channel, with which it connects and provides/controls Pitta in the arm. There are nineteen (19) pressure points (marmas) along this channel's trajectory. The energy flow direction is from the back of the little finger and along the back of the arm towards the trunk. Energy flows up

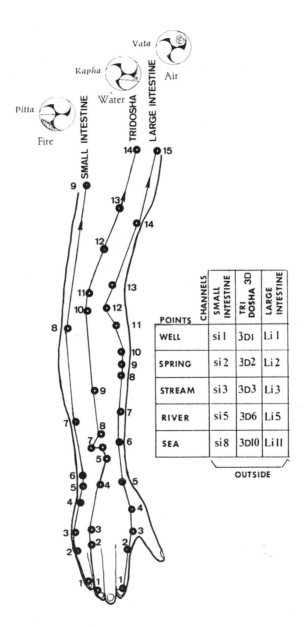

POINTS	CHANNELS	SMALL INTESTINE	TRI DOSHA 3D	LARGE INTESTINE
WELL		si 1	3DI	Li 1
SPRING		si 2	3D2	Li 2
STREAM		si 3	3D3	Li 3
RIVER		si 5	3D6	Li 5
SEA		si 8	3DI0	Li II

OUTSIDE

Fig. 22 Outside Arm Channels

the arm along the Small Intestine channel. The S.I. channel is a Pitta related channel in the arm along with the Heart channel.

Tridosha Channel (3D)

This channel connects with the Tridosha area of the body, which is a generalization of the three humors and its three sections of the trunk: Kapha (thorax), Pitta (below thorax and above navel) and Vata (below navel). The 3D channel therefore affects the mutual harmony of these three and the flow of fluids through these three areas. The 3D channel connects with the back of the ring finger and has twenty-three (23) marmas or needling points.

Large Intestine Channel (L.I.)

The Large Intestine channel is directly behind the Lung channel with which it is connected. There are twenty (20) pressure points (marmas) along the length of this channel. The flow of energy is from the index finger, up the arm to connect with the trunk. Marma numbering in this channel commences with LI.1 at the index finger.

INSIDE CHANNELS—Leg *(Antar Nadis)*

There are six channels on the leg, three are inside channels which means that they are solid organ channels and three are outside channels, which relate to the hollow organs (Fig. 23).

Spleen Channel (Sp)

The Spleen channel commences at the outside of the large toe and travels along the front aspect of the inside of the leg, then along the front of the body to reach the spleen. The energy flow direction in this organ channel is up the body. There are twenty one (21) pressure points (marmas) along the Spleen channel's trajectory, with Sp1 point being at the large toe. The Spleen channel connects with the Stomach channel from which it receives pranic energy.

Liver Channel (Lv)

The Liver channel commences at the inside of the large toe and travels upwards along the medial aspect of the inside of the leg, to

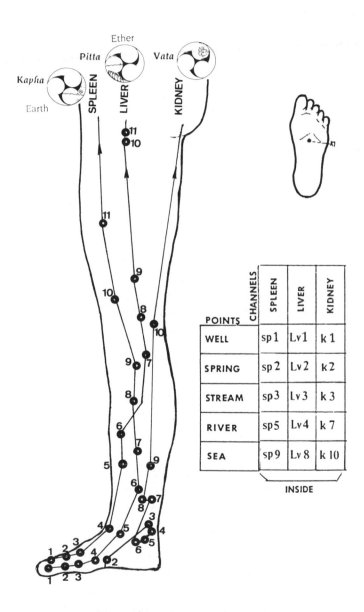

Fig. 23 Inside Leg Channels

POINTS	CHANNELS	SPLEEN	LIVER	KIDNEY
WELL		sp 1	Lv 1	k 1
SPRING		sp 2	Lv 2	k 2
STREAM		sp 3	Lv 3	k 3
RIVER		sp 5	Lv 4	k 7
SEA		sp 9	Lv 8	k 10

INSIDE

connect with the liver. There are fourteen (14) pressure points (marmas) along the Liver channel. The energy flow is up the body, from the large toe with Lv1 point being at the large toe. The Liver channel connects with the Gallbladder channel from which it receives pranic energy.

Kidney Channel (K)
The Kidney channel commences at the sole of the foot, travels up along the rear part of the inside of the leg, along the middle part of the front of the trunk, to conclude at the kidney. There are twenty-seven (27) pressure points (marmas) along this channel. The energy flow direction is up the body. The Kidney channel connects with the Urinary Bladder channel from which it receives its pranic energy.

OUTSIDE CHANNELS—Leg (Bahya Nadis)
The outside channels of the leg relate to the hollow organs below the diaphragm. They have the energy flow direction from the organs to the extremities (NOTE: opposite to the flow of energy of the same type of [outside] channels in the arm.)

Stomach Channel (St)
The Stomach channel commences at the middle of the bottom eyelid, travels down the cheek, then horizontally along the jaw , branching out later into (a) upwards towards the temple and (b) down from the jaw, along the side of the throat, directly down across the nipple and then parallel to the spine. It follows down the medial aspect of the front of the thigh to then conclude at the second toe. There are forty five (45) marmas or pressure points along its trajectory. The flow of energy direction is down towards the toes (Fig. 24).

Gallbladder Channel (Gb)
The Gallbladder channel starts at the corner of the eye, travels towards the ear, then travels up along the parietal area of the head, down along the back of the ear, the top of the shoulder, along the frontal costal and sacral areas, down the medial aspect of the outside of

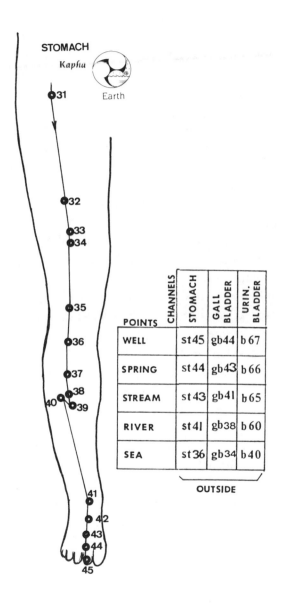

POINTS	CHANNELS	STOMACH	GALL BLADDER	URIN. BLADDER
WELL		st 45	gb 44	b 67
SPRING		st 44	gb 43	b 66
STREAM		st 43	gb 41	b 65
RIVER		st 41	gb 38	b 60
SEA		st 36	gb 34	b 40

OUTSIDE

Fig. 24 The Stomach (Outside Leg) Channel

the leg. The channel connects with the fourth toe (the one next to the small toe). There are forty four (44) marmas or pressure points along the Gallbladder channel with its flow of energy direction from the organ (Gb) down the leg (Fig. 25).

Urinary Bladder (Ub)

The Urinary Bladder channel (Fig. 26) commences next to the inside corner of the eye, travels along the center of the forehead, along the top and back of the head, down along the back of the body, parallel to and about two fingers width from the center of the spine (Fig. 27). The channel then follows down to the back of the knee. From there, it then continues by once again descending from the thoracic area, two fingers width parallel to the first section of the channel near the spine. It then reaches the back of the knee, down along the back of the leg to end up on the small toe.

There are sixty seven (67) marmas or pressure points along the Urinary Bladder channel with the flow of energy direction down the body, towards the toe.

It would appear logical that since the legs are longer than the arms, the number of points in the leg channels must be higher than the number of points in the arm channels.

Apparently, it was customary in the past to refer to channels according to their position (outside or inside of limb), leg or arm related and the humor which they represented. As an illustration, when referring to the Lung channel (solid, inside arm channel) it is called Antar Bahu Vata Nadi (Inside, Arm Vata Channel). The Large Intestine being an outside channel (because it is a hollow organ) is then referred to as Bahya Bahu Vata Nadi (Outside, Arm Vata Channel). Antar means "inside"; bahya means "outside"; bahu means "arm" and pada means "leg or foot".

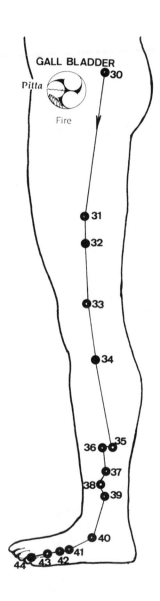

Fig. 25 The Gallbladder (Outside Leg) Channel

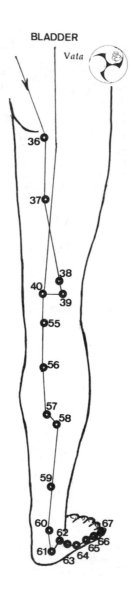

Fig. 26 The Urinary Bladder (Outside Leg) Channel

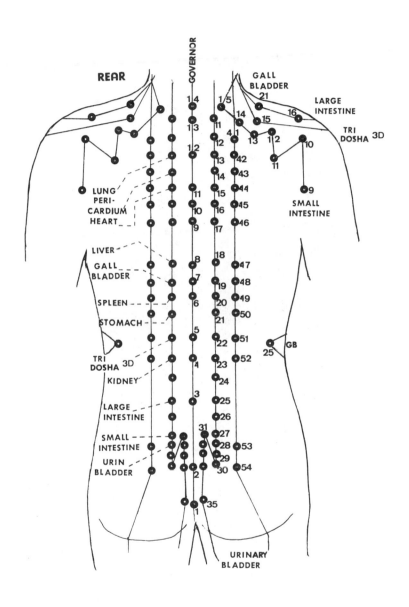

Fig. 27 The Channels on the rear of the body

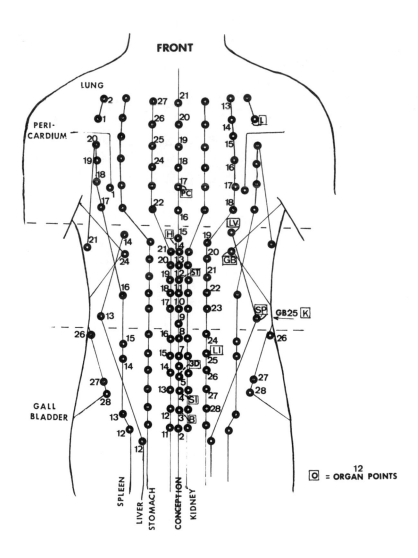

Fig. 28 The Channels on the front of the body

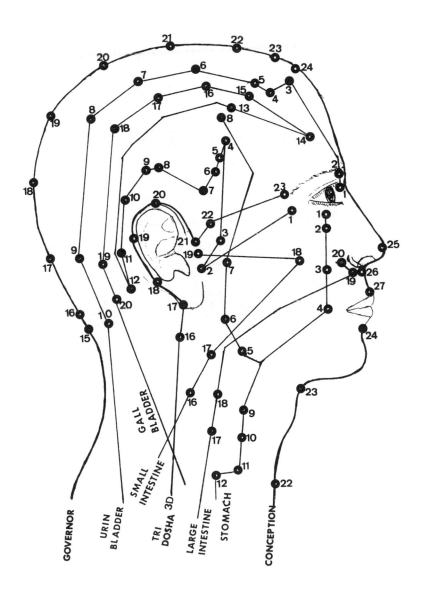

Fig. 29 The Channels on the head

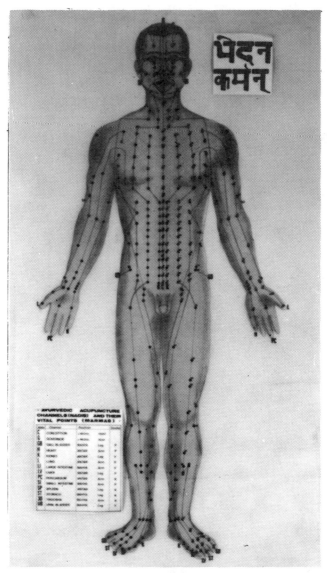

Front View

Fig. 30 Ayurvedic acupuncture channels (nadis)
and their vital points (marmas)

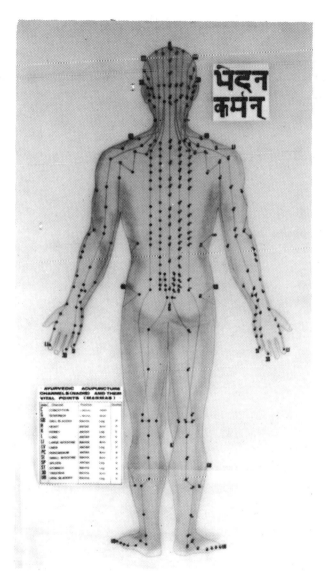

Rear View

Fig. 31

Channel Name	Position	Limb	Humor	
ARM				
Heart	Antar	Bahu	Pitta	Nadi
Small Intestine	Bahya	Bahu	Pitta	Nadi
Pericardium	Antar	Bahu	Kapha	Nadi
3D	Bahya	Bahu	Kapha	Nadi
Lung	Antar	Bahu	Vata	Nadi
Large Intestine	Bahya	Bahu	Vata	Nadi
LEG				
Liver	Antar	Pada	Pitta	Nadi
Gallbladder	Bahya	Pada	Pitta	Nadi
Spleen	Antar	Pada	Kapha	Nadi
Stomach	Bahya	Pada	Kapha	Nadi
Kidney	Antar	Pada	Vata	Nadi
U.Bladder	Bahya	Pada	Vata	Nadi

PART 3
VITAL POINTS
IMPORTANT MARMAS

The word marma means a sensitive spot which can be needled, massaged or heated in order to cause therapy, not only in the local area where the point is located, but also in related organs and remote areas which are connected together by the point's pranic channel. This interrelationship is due to mutual connections with Prana, the Five Elements and the three humors.

"These marma points are the seat of Prana."[3]

> *"Marma point is a concentrated point of Prana (energy). There are certain very vital anatomical points on the body surface which have secret and significant life values and they are composed of muscles, nerves, blood vessels, joints, ligaments and bones. Though it is not necessary that all [of these] structures should be present collectively at a time for the composition of marma, even if only two structures are present, it may constitute a marma point."*[4]

A marma is then a concentrated point of Prana, where several or all of the anatomical structures (muscle, bone, etc.) are also present. These points are connected like a pearl necklace by a common thread or channel called Nadi. The channel carries the energy to its related marmas.

Marmas connect with underlying channels which carry Prana or bio-energy. These channels lie deep in the body but occasionally they tend to wander towards the outside of the body. Where it does, it constitutes a marma, a low resistance area of the skin which has concentrated Prana. Sometimes these points become sensitive (painful) when touched or pressed, normally due to an imbalance in their related organ or if trauma has occurred around the area of the channel's trajectory. This is termed referred pain which is a reflex action, either local or remote.

141

LETHAL MARMAS

Other marmas are highly susceptible to a blow and therefore constitute the lethal marmas. There are approximately 107 of these, with some being more lethal than others, and when struck by a blow may result in death, coma, unconsciousness or delayed reactions which may cause disease. Normally, these lethal marmas are not needled in acupuncture.

> *"In classical acupuncture theory there are certain spots where it is prohibited to needle. These spots, and many more apparently not recorded by acupuncturists, when struck by a weapon, a fist or even a finger, will render the victim stunned, paralyzed, unconscious or dead."[5]*

These lethal points form the basis of those described by Charaka and Sushruta, since their consideration is important when performing surgery or when a patient is wounded at a marma site.

Traditionally, the location and methods of striking these lethal types of marmas have remained a closely guarded secret. No person in India was taught the lethal marma system until the prospective student had shown sufficient maturity and good character, and be a type most unlikely to abuse the system or teach others indiscriminately. The location of the marmas is only half of the knowledge necessary to be effective since some need to be hit, while are others are pinched or pressed in order to cause the required effect.

These 107 (or 108) lethal marmas are correlated by other experts in the Orient:

> *"Marma experts in South India have isolated 108 of these lethal spots. The locations of these vital points are extremely secret but we were able to check several well-known points with experts in Taiwan, South India and Japan, and there was almost complete agreement about their positions.*
>
> *Dr. Joseph Needham had the idea of checking with British forensic scientists about the likely consequences of striking some of these vital points. Their answers bore out exactly what he had been told by martial arts masters [in the Orient]."[6]*

ACUPUNCTURE MARMAS

The acupuncture points on the other hand are those which can be needled without any negative effect. There are literally hundreds of marmas in the body which can be needled in this way. As more research is done, new ones are continuously located and added to the repertoire. There are traditionally 180 major marmas in Ayurvedic acupuncture which can be used for treatment of almost any disease, since a disease is an imbalance in the energy field of the body. However, there are at least as many again which have minor but nevertheless important properties. As a result, there are at least 310 marmas from a traditional source, due to their connections with the organ channels. There are others like the lymphatic and allergy points on the hand which have evolved from modern research. Ayurvedic acupuncture, being a true system of needling, must continue research and expansion for the attainment of more knowledge, in parallel with any other system of acupuncture.

The pranic energy flow through the channels and anatomical positioning of the three humors in the body means that the closer the marma is to the organ, the more it relates to the physical aspect of the organ or the body. The further away it is found, the more subtle effect it will have on the body. For instance, treating Vata type symptoms of a subtle nature (nervousness, anxiety) can be treated by needling marma points further away from the trunk, in this case very near the end of the fingertips. Where the imbalance is of a more gross nature (e.g. physical damage to the heart muscle), then a point closer to the elbow is needled. Mental imbalances are normally of a Vata nature and are considered subtle. They too can be treated by points near the fingertips. Remembering that in the trunk, Vata is positioned below the navel (lowest area of the trunk), then it is clear that it too should be located near the fingertips or toes (lowest area of the limbs). Middle imbalances, like Pitta, are treated somewhere in between these two areas of the leg or arm, while Kapha is at the highest level of the trunk and limbs. (Fig. 32)

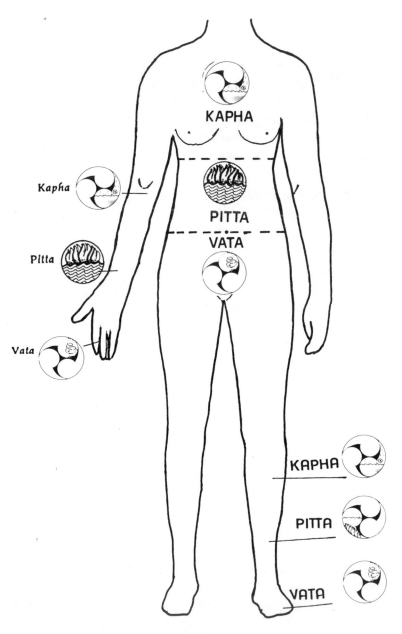

Fig. 32

An analogy can be drawn with electric conduction. Where a light or other electric device is close to the power source, it will normally have sufficient energy to allow it to function correctly. As the wire or cable is extended, this can, after a certain length, cause the light or device to malfunction or turn off because the current is now more subtle (there is less physical quantity). This does not mean that there is no current flow since if a smaller wattage globe is connected, it will shine brightly. The further away it is located from the power source, the less physical (lower wattage) transference of electricity into light the globe must be able to do.

Each solid and hollow organ channel on its own can not provide the necessary requirements for health, as there must be a solid organ in connection with a hollow one in accordance with the humors' functions and their locations in the body. Pitta in the arm for instance, cannot be achieved by simply the Heart channel on its own. The Small Intestine channel must also be there, since the organs' combination must be there for the humor's existence. When the solid and hollow organs combine, the humors function and therapy can be achieved by puncturing the appropriate related marmas or points.

Out of the most important points in acupuncture, there are some which are extremely important. These are the ones which directly relate to the Five Elements and connect with the 12 major organs via their channels. These are called the Five Element points (marmas). They are necessary for a true knowledge of Ayurvedic Acupuncture since the Five Elements are the nexus of Ayurveda and conjointly form the basis of the three humors.

FIVE ELEMENT POINTS (*Pancha Sru Marmas*)

The Five Elements of Fire, Earth, Wind, Water and Ether also appear as points along each of the channels, just as they appear in the five major chakras or nerve plexi. As there are five elements, Ayurveda similarly classifies five points in each channel and calls them the Five Flow Points (Pancha Sru Marmas). They are also sometimes referred to as the Pancha Bhautik Marmas (or Five Element points). The reason they are called flow points is because they relate to the flow of energy in much the same manner as water flows. Water is the element of flow.

Each organ channel in the body then has five points which reflect the Five Elements (e.g. in Heart, S.I., Lung channels, etc.). They appear in each channel according to a particular format which is always the Wheel of Support and its exclusive connection between the Five Elements.

The sequence of appearance differs between the solid organ channels and the hollow organ channels. All solid organ channels have Ether as the first element points, with each subsequent one being according to the Wheel of Support i.e. — Ether, Fire, Earth, Wind, Water. The first element marma is thus Ether, the fifth or last is therefore Water.

All hollow organs have, instead, Wind as their first element points, with each subsequent one being according to the same wheel i.e. Wind, Water, Ether, Fire and Earth.

The reason for the difference in elements between these two types of organ channels is clearly seen when we truly realize why the element points are positioned where they are. The connection between the hollow and solid organ channels via the element points allows the creation of the humors and their treatment thereof. By this is meant that the mutual connection between each similar point along each channel affects the humors (Fig. 33).

Vata

Take, for instance, the first points of both the solid and the hollow organ channels. Without a doubt, the channels' connections is due to a common element (e.g. Large Intestine/Lung by Wind) but the first marma on each of the two organ channels relate to Ether (in the solid organ channel) and Wind (in the hollow organ channel). This connection of the two elements at these two points forms the Ayurvedic most subtle humor called Vata which is composed of Wind and

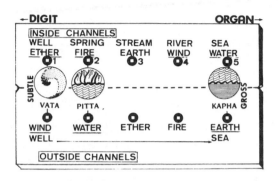

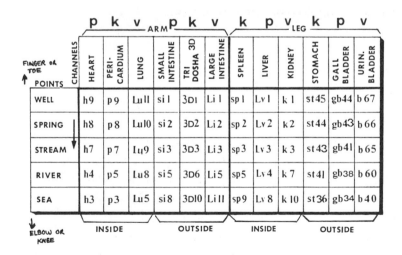

FINGER OR TOE ↑ POINTS	CHANNELS	HEART	PERI-CARDIUM	LUNG	SMALL INTESTINE	TRI DOSHA 3D	LARGE INTESTINE	SPLEEN	LIVER	KIDNEY	STOMACH	GALL BLADDER	URIN. BLADDER
WELL		h9	p9	Lu11	si1	3D1	Li1	sp1	Lv1	k1	st45	gb44	b67
SPRING		h8	p8	Lu10	si2	3D2	Li2	sp2	Lv2	k2	st44	gb43	b66
STREAM		h7	p7	Lu9	si3	3D3	Li3	sp3	Lv3	k3	st43	gb41	b65
RIVER		h4	p5	Lu8	si5	3D6	Li5	sp5	Lv4	k7	st41	gb38	b60
SEA		h3	p3	Lu5	si8	3D10	Li11	sp9	Lv8	k10	st36	gb34	b40

ELBOW OR KNEE   INSIDE   OUTSIDE   INSIDE   OUTSIDE

Fig. 33 The Five Flow Points and humors relationships

Ether. These, of course, are the two most subtle elements.

Pitta

The second set of points along each of the two types of channels relate to Pitta, since one is the Fire element point (solid organ channel) while the other is the Water element (hollow organ channel) and Pitta is created out of Fire and Water.

Kapha

The last or fifth points are Water, in the solid organ channels and Earth, in the hollow organ channels. This equates with Kapha which is the most physical humor out of the three and which itself is composed of Earth and Water, the two most physical elements. As can be seen, their total interrelationship results in the continuation of the three humors in the body via connection of the two types of organ channels (solid and hollow).

Points	Solid Organs	Hollow Organs	Humor
1st	Ether	Wind	VATA
2nd	Fire	Water	PITTA
3rd	Earth	Ether	
4th	Wind	Fire	
5th	Water	Earth	KAPHA

The outline of the elements mentioned directly above will also demonstrate a second wheel of the elements in action, that is, the Wheel of Creation where one element leads to the creation of another. This is usually as follows: Ether, Wind, Fire, Water and Earth. Studying the above, it will be noticed that within the five pairs of points, there is a "threading" between the solid organ channels and the hollow organ channels according to the Wheel of Creation. It appears to occur twice, starting at the solid organ element Ether, following through directly across to Wind, diagonally down to Fire, then across to Water, diagonally across to Earth and then directly across to Ether before the cycle commences again at the 4th set of points.

The combination of the first set of points (hollow/solid channels) as previously explained, results in Vata. These two points (Ether-Wind) may nevertheless be needled for problems relating to mental illness or subtle imbalances like Vata.

The combination of the second set of points results in the formation of Pitta (Fire-Water). These two points are usually indicated in febrile diseases (Pitta).

The combination of the third set of points does not create a separate humor in this case but the points are indicated in painful disorders of the joints, especially those of a Kapha (Earth) type.

The fourth set of points is usually indicated in respiratory disorders due to their Wind connection.

The combination of the fifth set of points, (Earth and Water in both types of channels) results in the formation of Kapha (Earth-Water). These points are usually indicated in physical disorders of the organs themselves, just as Kapha is the most physical of the three humors.

Ancients noticed long ago that water evaporates, rises and forms clouds. It is this same water that falls from the clouds during rain, and collects on the ground to subsequently find its way to the sea. Ayurveda realized that there is a difference between cloud (evaporated) water and water found on the earth. This difference is Prana and nutrients. When water falls from the clouds, it collects Prana but it has no nutrients. As the water runs along the ground (e.g. stream or river), it picks up nutrients like minerals which are necessary for the body. So the concept of the flow of water is that it commences on a very subtle level (it only has Prana) and then gradually becomes more physical as nutrients are added to it. The Five Elements also reflect this same subtle to physical path of Prana, and traditionally each of the five points were labelled with a name reminiscent to the flow of water.

Consequently, the first set of points deals with the subtle aspect of the flow of Prana, that is, the Vata humor, and the two subtle elements of Ether and Wind. Due to this, these first points are generically termed the Well points for easier identification. When the Well point is needled, that could indicate either Ether or Wind are involved with the solid or hollow organ channels. The term "well" is according to the natural process by which water falls to the ground, collecting Prana from the atmosphere as it does. It forms a small well before enough water can collect there to spill and flow elsewhere. The Well point is somewhat like the Ether element, the first of the Five Elements and the most subtle.

The second set of points are collectively or singularly referred to as the Spring points, since a spring is the next level of water flow. This is reminiscent of the Wind element, the second element along the Wheel of Creation according to its attributes.

The third set is referred to as the Stream points, a somewhat larger effect (more physical) than the previous two sets of points, much like the effect of the Fire element.

The fourth set of points is the River, since like the Water element, it is the second most physical structure.

This finally empties into the sea. These last two points are consequently referred to as the Sea points, where the effect is the most physical, much like the Earth element and Kapha.

The concept of the terminology and philosophy of the five points: Well, Spring, Stream, River and Sea is therefore analogous with the appearance of the elements according to the Wheel of Creation. The actual elements located in these points are nevertheless according to the Wheel of Support, starting with the most subtle: Ether for the solid organ channels and Wind for the hollow organ channels. As a result, the Well points deal with Vata, the most subtle; the Spring points deal with Pitta, the middle humor and the Sea points deal with Kapha, the most physical of the three humors. The Sea tends to contain more water than any of the others and thus it is also more physical (like Kapha).

The Well, Spring, Stream, River and Sea points are also on a par with the stages of disease according to Ayurveda, previously explained.

- The Well points are related to Aggravation,
- Spring points with Overflow,
- Stream points with Displacement,
- River points with Manifestation and the
- Sea points with Flowering—the last stage and most physical of all five.

PARENT-CHILD *(Pitar-Bala)*

Each of the five points described above are in essence a reflection of the Five Elements and their related humors and organs. Treatment of an organ (affecting a humor) is carried out according to the concept of a parent-child, another ancient observation of nature, which affects the Five Elements. The Parent-Child concept utilizes the Wheel of Support of the Five Elements and describes the method where an unbalanced element is treated by needling organs or points relative to it, according to the natural process of feeding (or supporting). The parent is responsible for feeding the child; the child is responsible for taking the food from the parent. Where the mother has an excess in breast milk, a simple remedy is to allow the baby to feed. This has the effect of emptying the breast of milk.

Where a baby is *deficient* in food (is hungry), the parent is encouraged to feed the child. This explains the Parent-Child concept which can be used to increase energy in an organ/element by treating the element's parent (encouraging the parent to feed the child) or by decreasing an excess of energy in the element/organ by treating the element's child (encouraging the child to feed from the parent).

According to the Wheel of Support,

- Ether is the parent of Fire but also the child of Water.
- Fire is the parent of Earth, but the child of Ether.
- Earth is the parent of Wind, but the child of Fire.
- Wind is the parent of Water, but the child of Earth and
- Water is the parent of Ether but the child of Wind.

An excess of energy in the Water element (kidney/bladder) for instance, can be reduced by treating this element's child (Ether).

A deficiency of energy in the Water element can be increased by treating this element's parent (Wind). This concept applies to all the other elements according to the Wheel of Support.

Treatment of the elements/organs can be performed on the appropriate element point according to the Parent-Child concept. Treatment of the humors can be carried out by needling the set of points which reflect the vitiated humor, that is: Well points for Vata, Spring points for Pitta and Sea points for Kapha.

TREATMENT

Acupuncture treatment of the humors can be performed by treating the corresponding organ channels, that is, those related to the humors (listed in the Bio-energy clock or Pranic Mandala Fig. 5). Treatment of the appropriate Five Sru points (Fig. 33) can similarly affect the humors. For example, a Vata imbalance is treated by needling the Well points of the related organ channels of Large Intestine and Lung (arm) or Kidney and Bladder (leg). If an imbalance is located along a particular limb, then the related humoral channels in that locale are utilized; (e.g. Lung/L.I. for Vata in the arm).

Pitta can be similarly treated by needling the Spring points of the Pitta related channels. Kapha can be treated by needling the Sea points of the appropriate Kapha channels. In theory, since all channels connect together in a loop, then any two related channels' Well points can be needled to treat a vitiated humor. However, in practice, the corresponding channels may offer a faster, better alternative.

Chronological

Treatment should also be carried out with special consideration of the time of day or night with regards to the type of imbalance. Each vitiated humor reacts best to treatments carried out during the humor's risk times, according to the Pranic Mandala. Kapha is best treated during Kapha times, Pitta during Pitta's times and Vata, during Vata's risk times.

Where an element is either in excess or deficiency, treatment according to the Mandala is also appropriate. An element in excess should be treated just prior to the organ's energy peak of pranic energy, while a deficiency is best treated directly after the peak of pranic energy of the organ.

Chronological-related treatment of diseases is not always possible today in the West, unless carried out in a proper hospital setting, where the patient is available on a twenty-four hour basis. Private clinics have certain hours of business and are not always available at the times the patient may require the chronological treatment. Nevertheless, treatment of channels during business hours (between 9 a.m. - 5 p.m.) will still provide a means of healing and, although not ideal, is quite effective.

OTHER IMPORTANT POINTS

As well as the Five Sru Points, there are some other points which perform special functions.

Bridge (Connector) Points *(Setu Marmas)*

There are some points which connect between the hollow and solid organ channels and allow Prana to travel between one channel and the next in line. Each channel has one of these connecting points between the hollow and solid organ channels. The Vata in the arm consists of the Lung and Large Intestine channels. These two are linked together by a connecting point located in each of these two channels. The use of the connecting point enhances the therapeutic value of the treatment. The Lung channel's Bridge point is Lung 7 (L7) while the Large Intestine channel's Bridge point is LI 6, so their needling will assist Vata type problems (or imbalances in the lungs or large intestine). The connecting points are normally referred to as Bridge points and are termed "Setu Marmas." They demonstrate the existence of a nadi (a bridge) between the two related channels.

Source Points *(Mula Marmas)*

Source points (Mula Marmas) are points where Prana tends to be retained in the channel and forms a type of base. The word "Mula" actually means root or base. These points tend to reinforce the therapeutic effect by balancing energy in the channel or organ which is unbalanced.

Channels	Source Points	Bridge Points	
Heart	* H7	H5	(H-SI)
Pericardium	* P7	P6	(P-3D)
Lung	* L9	L7	(L-LI)
Small Intestine	SI4	SI7	(SI-H)
Tridosha	3D4	3D5	(3D-P)
Large Intestine	LI4	LI6	(LI-L)
Liver	* Lv3	Lv5	(Lv-GB)
Spleen	* Sp3	Sp4	(Sp-St)
Kidney	* K3	K4	(K-UB)
Gallbladder	GB40	GB37	(GB-Lv)
Stomach	St42	St40	(St-Sp)
Bladder	UB64	UB58	(UB-K)

The Source marmas or points with asterisks (*) in the above chart are also Stream points of the Five Elements in the solid organ channels.

PART 4
TREATMENT OF THE FIVE TRIDOSHAS

Ayurvedic medicine considers that each Vata, Pitta and Kapha can be further divided into five groups, each in accordance with their effects and functions in the body. Essentially, all humors are different polarities of Prana and have acquired different characteristics as they travel through the body. Each element is represented by one Vata, one Pitta and one Kapha and the element's effect on the body is mirrored by the appropriate humors (Fig. 34).

ETHER *(Inward-Controlling Effect)*
The Ether element relates to the functions of inward movement and controlling effects in the body and is represented by:
(1) Prana Vayu (Vata). Positioned in the brain, this one has the directing effect on the other Vatas, and consequently is involved in most diseases. Acupuncture can directly treat diseases via this type of Prana, which also governs the correct functions of swallowing, belching, inhalation and sneezing.
(2) Sadhaka Pitta. Centered in the brain and the heart it controls the subtle intellect, since Ether is the most subtle of the Five Elements. Fantasies and reality become indistinguishable when this Pitta becomes vitiated.
(3) Tarpaka Kapha. This is also in the brain and heart (cerebro-spinal fluid) due to its connection with the subtle Ether, but being Kapha, it lubricates these parts of the body to give mental stability and correct memory recollection, the grounding feature of Kapha.

WIND *(Upward Movement)*
The Wind element relates to moving air and upward movements and is represented by:
(1) Udana Vayu (Vata). Positioned in the lung (chest and throat),

155

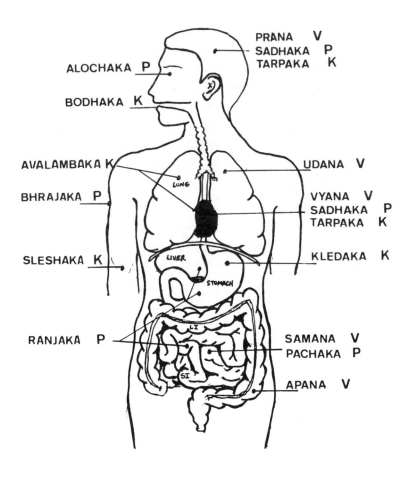

Fig. 34 The Five forms of Vata, Pitta and Kapha
and their locations

this Vayu controls exhalation and speech. Its vitiation may result in belching, coughs and vomiting. The connection with Vata, the Wind element and the lungs becomes quite obvious.

(2) Alochaka Pitta. This Pitta in connection with the Wind element allows the subtle reception of minute light particles via the eyes (Pitta sense organ). It is positioned in the eyes and its malfunction may result in failure of vision.

(3) Bodhaka Kapha. It is found in the mouth and affects the sense of taste, while its vitiation causes a lack of taste. Its connection with the Wind element ties it down to the respiratory system of which the mouth and tongue are part. Its derangement (as in too much Wind evaporating Water) results in a lack of taste since water is needed for tasting.

FIRE *(Digestive Process)*

The Fire element relates to transformation of things (digestion) and is represented by:

(1) Samana Vayu (Vata). This is found in the small intestine and controls the digestion. Its connection with Wind means it is the mover of the digestive system, while its vitiation can cause indigestion or lack of appetite.

(2) Pachaka Pitta. This is also located in the small intestine and supports the other forms of Pitta. It aids circulation, regulates body temperature and assists in the digestion of food. When deranged, it will cause heat to rise- e.g.hyperacidity, ulcers, etc.

(3) Kledaka Kapha. This is found in the stomach (and the alkaline secretions in the mucous lining of the digestive tract) and is responsible for the first stage of digestion.

WATER *(Diffusion/Distribution Process)*

The Water element relates to the process of distribution and diffusion and is represented by:

(1) Vyana Vayu (Vata). This is found in the heart and is distributed throughout the body due to its connection with Water and the active element Wind (Vayu). It lubricates the joints and muscles, thus con-

trolling their movements. As the kidneys (Water) are found in the lower part of the trunk, Vyana Vayu mainly affects the legs and their movements.

(2) Bhrajaka Pitta. This is found on the skin and maintains the skin's color and complexion, controlling warmth and light into the body. When vitiated, it causes rashes and discoloration of the skin.

(3) Sleshaka Kapha. This is located in the synovial fluid of the joints, due to its strong connection not only to Kapha but also to the Water element. When deranged, joint looseness and heaviness will occur.

EARTH *(Downward Movement—Stability)*

The Earth element relates to the downward movements of the body and its stability and is represented by:

(1) Apana Vayu (Vata). This is in the large intestine and controls all downward movement of elimination, urination, parturition, sex and menstruation. This is because of Earth's heavy, falling tendency and connection with Vata, which is positioned in the trunk area in which all of the controlling organs of these functions are to be found (e.g. kidney, L.I. sexual organs.)

(2) Ranjaka Pitta. This is found in the small intestine, stomach, liver and spleen and gives their related secretions their color and texture (e.g. to the bile, stool and urine). When deranged, it strongly colors these secretions.

(3) Avalambaka Kapha. This is found in the lung and the heart and gives correct lubrication to the chest area, since it relates to Earth (a Kapha element) and to the upper most area of the trunk (relating to Kapha). Due to this, it is possibly the most important form of Kapha when treating a patient. Some believe this corresponds to plasma, which is distributed by the heart and lungs.

Treatment

Each of the above forms can be treated by utilizing the correct organ channel as well as the appropriate points which affect the vitiated humor.

NAME	ORGAN	CHANNEL	POINTS
ETHER			
Vata—Prana	Brain	Heart/S.I.	Well
Pitta—Sadhaka	Brain/heart	Heart/S.I.	Spring
Kapha—Tarpaka	Brain/heart	Heart/S.I.	Sea
WIND			
Vata—Udana	Lung/chest	Lung/L.I.	Well
Pitta—Alochaka	Eyes	Lung/L.I.	Spring
Kapha—Bodhaka	Mouth/tongue	Lung/L.I.	Sea
FIRE			
Vata—Samana	S.Intestine	S.I./Heart	Well
Pitta—Pachaka	S.Intestine	S.I./Heart	Spring
Kapha—Kledaka	S.Intestine	S.I./Heart	Sea
WATER			
Vata—Vyana	Heart/body	3D/Pericard.	Well
Pitta—Bhrajaka	Skin	3D/Pericard.	Spring
Kapha—Sleshaka	Synovial	3D/Pericard.	Sea (arm joints)
		Kid/Blad.	Sea (leg joints)
EARTH			
Vata—Apana	L.Intestine	L.I./Lung	Well (arm)
		Kid./Bladder	Well (leg)
Pitta—Ranjaka	Lv.Sp.St.S.I.	Spleen/Stom.	Spring
Kapha–Avalambaka	Heart/lung	3D/Pericard.	Sea

NOTES:
1. *Science and Secrets of Early Medicine,* p. 211
2. *Light on Pranayama,* p. 32
3. *Acupuncture Marma and ther Asian therapeutic techniques,* p. 5
4. *Ibid.,* p. 15
5. *The Way of the Warrior,* p. 106
6. *Ibid.,* p. 107

CONCLUSION

Ayurveda is the "Science of Life," a lofty term that totally embodies this sophisticated and ancient system of medicine. However, due to certain factors in India, this science began to be fractionalized and consequently was almost destroyed.

The knowledge or information which has remained has been carefully protected and nurtured by family inheritance and in many cases by those who were brave enough to risk their own lives for its continuation. These people also had other knowledge to protect besides the medical sciences, so that the keepers of the knowledge of Indian martial arts also zealously defended this powerful knowledge of medicine. It is not a strange coincidence therefore that masters of Indian martial arts today are for the most part also highly skilled doctors of Ayurveda. In fact, Charaka himself stated that Ayurvedic medical knowledge is not only to be practised by doctors but also "by kshatriyas [warriors] for protection." (p. 503), (*Charaka Samhitta-Sutrasthana XXX*).

Like the martial art systems of Kalari and Marma Adi, Ayurvedic Acupuncture has remained cloaked in secrecy and unknown to the general populace. It has been traditionally conveyed from parent to child through word-of-mouth and kept within families.

The Ayurvedic Acupuncture system, like Ayurveda itself, is based on and takes refuge in the knowledge of Prana, the life-force, and in the Five Elements which originate from Prana. In the human body, these six natural factors give rise to the Tridoshas, the three Ayurvedic biological forces or humours. These nine factors also have direct effects on more physical entities like the organs and tissues so that their interrelationships are well charted. Each major organ has an energy channel (nadi) which is positioned along a limb and the trunk, and which contains a number of pressure or reflex points (marmas) along its length. These points can be needled, heated or massaged to cause a balancing effect on the energy which then results in health (homoeostasis). This is why Indian Acupuncture is correctly termed Ayurvedic Acupuncture because it utilizes Ayurvedic principles.

A point of synthesis must be established between what is popularly practised and that which is kept reserved, between the practical (in a remote clinic) and the academic (as taught in universities and used in hospitals). It is only in placing acupuncture in a practical, academic form that its continuation, propagation and expansion will be ensured. Its cloistered form today no longer serves a useful purpose; in fact it could serve as its epitaph.

This book should provide the basis to stimulate further research and interest in an important branch of possibly the most ancient and comprehensive medical system in the world. It requires much effort on the part of other Ayurvedic researchers to enhance and expand it so as to create a source of continuity for the present and future health of the human race.

APPENDIX A

MAJOR MARMAS AND THEIR THERAPEUTIC EFFECTS

MAJOR ARM POINTS

Key: P. = Perpendicular puncture
O. = Obliquely
H. = Horizontally
Number e.g. 15 mm = maximum depth of puncture (e.g. P. 15mm) = puncture perpendicularly to a depth maximum of 15mm.

LUNG CHANNEL

ELEMENT—Wind
ORGAN—Lung   **TYPE:** Solid Organ
HUMOR—Vata (Primary)
TIME OF ENERGY PEAK—3-5 a.m.
CHANNEL LOCATION—Inside of Arm (near thumb)

L.11 (WELL)—Ether
Cough, sore throat, nosebleed, asthma, febrile diseases, loss of consciousness, mental disorders. O. 4mm

L.10 (SPRING)—Fire
Cough, asthma, fever, spitting of blood, sore throat, pharyngitis. P. 15mm

L.9 (STREAM and SOURCE)—Earth
Cough, sore throat, asthma, spitting of blood, pain in chest and medial aspect of lung, palpitations. P. 8mm

L.8 (RIVER)—Wind
Cough, sore throat, asthma, pain in chest and wrist. P. 6mm

L.7 (BRIDGE POINT)
Cough, headache, neck rigidity, sore throat, asthma, facial paralysis, trismus, weakness of wrist. O. 12.5mm

L.6. (CLEFT POINT)
Cough, sore throat, tonsillitis, asthma, spitting of blood, elbow and arm pain and motor impairment. P. 15mm

L.5. (SEA POINT)—WATER
Cough, fever in p.m., spitting of blood, asthma, sore throat, pharyngitis, fullness in chest, spasmodic pain in elbow and arm. P. 12.5mm

L.4.
Pain in the middle of the arm, chest fullness and cough. P. 12.5mm

L.3.
Pain in the middle of the arm, nosebleed and asthma. P. 12.5mm

L.2.
Chest pain, shoulder pain, pain in chest, backache, asthma and cough. P. 25mm

L.1. (Lung front organ point)
Chest pain, shoulder and arm pain, fullness of chest, asthma and cough. P. 12.5mm

PERICARDIUM CHANNEL

ELEMENT—Water

ORGAN—Pericardium   TYPE: Solid Organ
HUMOR—Kapha (Secondary)
TIME OF ENERGY PEAK—7-9 p.m.
CHANNEL LOCATION—Medical aspect of inside of Arm

P.9. (WELL)—Ether
Cardiac pain, heat stroke, irritability, febrile diseases, loss of consciousness, aphasia with stiffness of tongue, sensation of fever in palm, convulsion in children. 0. 4mm

P.8. (SPRING)—Fire
Cardiac pain, mental disorders, vomiting, halitosis, epilepsy, stomatitis, hand and foot fungal infection. P. 12.5mm

P.7. (STREAM and SOURCE)—Earth
Cardiac pain, palpitation , mental disorders, vomiting, panic, epilepsy, gastric pain, pain in the chest and hypochondriac region. P. 12.5mm

P.6 (BRIDGE POINT)
Cardiac pain, palpitation, mental disorders, malaria, epilepsy, febrile diseases, gastric pains, vomiting, arm and elbow pain and contracture. P. 25mm

P.5 (RIVER)—Wind
Cardiac pain, palpitation, mental disorders, febrile diseases, irritability, malaria, gastric pain, vomiting, mental disorders, epilepsy, swelling of axilla, twitching and contracture of elbow, arm pain. P. 25mm

P.4 (CLEFT)
Cardiac pain, palpitation, angina pectoris, nosebleed, furuncle, vomiting of blood. P. 20mm

P.3 (SEA)—Water
Cardiac pain, febrile diseases, irritability, palpitations, gastric pain, vomiting, elbow and arm pain, hand and arm tremors. P. 20mm

P.2
Cardiac pain, chest pain, pain in upper arm, cough. P. 15mm

P.1
Axillary swelling and pain, pain in hypochondria, feeling of suffocation in chest. 0. 6mm

HEART CHANNEL

ELEMENT—Fire
ORGAN—Heart   TYPE: Solid Organ
HUMOR—Pitta (Primary)
TIME OF ENERGY PEAK—11am-1pm
CHANNEL LOCATION—Inside of arm (little finger side)

H.9 (WELL)—Ether
Cardiac pain, mental disorders, palpitations, unconsciousness, febrile diseases, pain in chest and hypochondriac region. 0. 4mm

H.8. (SPRING)—Fire
Palpitation, chest pain, twitching and contracture of little finger, feverish sensation in palm, enuresis, skin pruritus, dysuria. P. 12.5mm

H.7 (STREAM and SOURCE)—Earth
Cardiac pain, insomnia, mental disorders, irritability, palpitation, hysteria, poor memory, epilepsy, yellow sclera, pain in the hypochondria, sensation of fever in palm. P. 12.5mm

H.6 (CLEFT POINT)
Cardiac pain, night sweating, hysteria. P. 12.5mm

H.5 (BRIDGE POINT)
Palpitation, hysteria, blurring of vision, sore throat, dizziness, sudden hoarseness, aphasia (with stiffness in tongue), pain in wrist and arm, angina pectoris. P. 12.5mm

H.4 (RIVER)—Wind
Cardiac pain, convulsions, sudden hoarseness, contracture of elbow and arm. P. 12.5mm

H.3 (SEA)—Water
Cardiac pain, tremors in hand, numbness of arm, contracture of elbow, pain in axilla and hypochondriac region, primary tuberculosis of cervical lymph nodes (scrofula) P. 12.5mm

H.2
Hypochondriac, shoulder and arm pains, yellow sclera. P. 12.5mm

H.1
Pain in side and heart regions, elbow and arm coldness and pain, primary tuberculosis of the cervical lymph nodes (scrofula) P. 25mm

LARGE INTESTINE CHANNEL

ELEMENT—Wind
ORGAN—Large Intestine   **TYPE:** Solid Organ
HUMOR—Vata (Primary)
TIME OF ENERGY PEAK—5-7 a.m.
CHANNEL LOCATION—Thumb side of outside of arm.

LI.1 (WELL)—Wind
Sore throat, submandibular area swelling, toothache, finger numbness, febrile disease, loss of consciousness. 0. 4mm

LI.2 (SPRING)—Water
Nosebleed, blurring of vision, toothache, sore throat, pharyngitis, febrile disease, backache. P. 8mm

LI.3 (STREAM)—Ether
Toothache, pain in the eye, sore throat, redness and swelling of the fingers and dorsum of hand. P. 25mm

LI.4 (SOURCE)
Toothache, headache, redness / swelling and pain in the eye, facial swelling, sore throat, nosebleed, motor disturbance of the trigeminal nerve, facial paralysis, febrile disease without perspiration, hidrosis, amenorrhea, delayed labor, abdominal pain, dysentery, constipation. P. 20mm

LI.5 (RIVER)—Fire
Toothache, headache, sore throat, redness with swelling and pain of the eye, wrist pain. P. 12.5mm

LI.6 (BRIDGE POINT)
Deafness, aching of hand and arm, nosebleed, edema. P. 12.5mm

LI.7 (CLEFT POINT)
Headache, sore throat, abdominal noises, abdominal pain, aching of shoulder and arm, facial swelling. P. 20mm

LI.8
Pain in abdominal area and the elbow and arm. P. 15mm

LI.9
Pain in the abdominal area, hand and arm numbness, arm and head motor impairment, shoulder ache, abdominal noises. P. 25mm

LI.10
  Head and arm motor impairment, vomiting, diarrhea, abdominal and shoulder pain. P. 25mm

LI.11 (SEA POINT)—Earth
  Head and arm motor impairment, sore throat, tonsillitis, fever, urticaria, goiter, vomiting, diarrhea, dysentery, primary tuberculosis of cervical lymph nodes (scrofula), elbow, shoulder and arm pain, high blood pressure. P. 25mm

LI.12
  Elbow and arm numbness and pain. P. 12.5mm

LI.13
  Primary tuberculosis of cervical lymph nodes (scrofula), elbow and arm pain. P. 12.5mm

LI.14
  Scrofula, head and arm motor impairment, arm and shoulder pain, backache, eye disease. P. 12.5mm

LI.15
  Scrofula, head and arm motor impairment, arm and shoulder pain, german measles. O. 25mm (down the arm)

LI.16
  Head and arm pain and motor impairment, shoulder pain. P. 15mm

LI.17
  Scrofula, enlargement of the thyroid gland (goiter), hoarse and sore throat. P. 12.5mm

LI.18
  Scrofula, enlargement of the thyroid gland (goiter), hoarse and sore throat, expectoration, asthma, cough. P. 12.5mm

LI.19
  Nasal obstruction, mouth deviation, nose bleed. O. 8mm

LI.20
  Nasal obstruction, mouth deviation, nosebleed, runny nose, facial swelling and itch, gastric region pain. O. 8mm

TRIDOSHA (3D) CHANNEL

ELEMENT—Water
ORGAN—Tridosha (3D)   **TYPE**—**Hollow Organ**
HUMOR—Kapha (Secondary)
TIME OF ENERGY PEAK—9-11 p.m.
CHANNEL LOCATION—Medial aspect of outside of arm

3D.1 (WELL)—Wind
  Headaches, irritability, febrile diseases, redness of eyes, sore throat, stiffness of tongue. O. 4mm

3D.2 (SPRING)—Water
  Headache, deafness, malaria, redness of eyes, sore throat, pain in hand and arm. O. 12.5mm

3D.3 (STREAM)—Ether
  Headache, febrile diseases, tinnitus, deafness, redness of eyes, sore throat, pain in elbow and arm, motor impairment of fingers. P. 12.5mm

3D.4 (SOURCE)
  Malaria, deafness, wrist/shoulder and arm pain. P. 8mm

3D.5 (BRIDGE POINT)
  Headaches, febrile diseases, deafness, cheek and hypochondria pains, tinnitus, elbow and arm motor impairment, pain in fingers, hand tremors, arthritis in arm. P. 25mm

3D.6 (RIVER)—Fire
Tinnitus, deafness, sudden hoarseness, heavy sensation and aches of shoulder and back, constipation and vomiting. P. 25mm

3D.7 (CLEFT)
Epilepsy, deafness, pain in upper extremity. P. 25mm

3D.8
Deafness, sudden voice hoarseness, arm and hand pains. P. 25mm

3D.9
Deafness, toothache, sudden voice hoarseness, forearm pain. P. 25mm

3D.10 (SEA)—Earth
Epilepsy, one sided headaches. P. 12.5mm

3D.11
Shoulder and arm pains. P. 8mm

3D.12
Neck and arm pains, stiffness of neck, headache. P. 15mm

3D.13
Swelling of the thyroid gland (goiter), arm and shoulder pains. P. 20mm

3D.14
Arm pain, heaviness in shoulder. P. 25mm (down arm)

3D.15
Neck, shoulder and arm pains, neck stiffness. P. 12.5mm

3D.16
Swelling of the facial area, dizziness, blurred vision, rigidity in neck, deafness of a sudden nature. P. 12.5mm

3D.17
Swelling of the cheek area, deafness, ringing in the ears, paralysis of the face, motor disturbance of the trigeminal nerve. P. 25mm

3D.18
Ringing in the ears, deafness, headaches. O. 4mm

3D.19
Earache, ringing in the ears , headaches. O. 4mm

3D.20
Toothache, eye and ear redness and swelling, eye pain. O. 4mm (down)

3D.21
Toothache, ringing in the ears, deafness, discharge from ear. P. 12.5mm

3D.22
Lockjaw, heaviness and ache in head, ringing in the ears. O. 8mm

3D.23
Twitching of the eyelid, headache, blurred vision, eye redness and pain. P. 8mm

SMALL INTESTINE CHANNEL

ELEMENT—Fire
ORGAN—Small Intestine   **TYPE:** Hollow Organ
HUMOR—Pitta (+Agni) (Primary)
TIME OF ENERGY PEAK—1-3 p.m.
CHANNEL LOCATION—Little finger aspect of outside of arm

SI.1 (WELL)—Wind
Febrile diseases, loss of consciousness, cornea cloudiness, sore throat, deficiency in lactation. O. 4mm

SI.2 (SPRING)—Water
Febrile diseases, finger numbness. P. 8mm

SI.3 (STREAM)—Ether
Febrile diseases, epilepsy, malaria, headache, night sweating, rigidity of neck, deafness, eye congestion, backache, contracture and twitching of elbow, arm and fingers. P. 15mm

SI.4 (SOURCE)
Febrile diseases, headaches, jaundice, neck rigidity, cornea cloudiness, pain in hypochondria. P. 12.5mm

SI.5 (RIVER)—Fire
Febrile diseases, neck and submandibular swelling, wrist and lateral arm pain. P. 10mm

SI.6 (CLEFT)
Blurred vision, hysteria, arm arthritis, shoulder, back, arm and elbow aches. P. 12.5mm

SI.7 (BRIDGE POINT)
Febrile diseases, mental disorders, neck rigidity, contracture and twisting of elbow, finger pain. P. 12.5mm

SI.8 (SEA)—Earth
Epilepsy, swelling of cheek, pain in nape and in the side rear area of shoulder and arm. P. 15mm

SI.9
Tinnitus, deafness, hand and arm motor impairment and pain, pain in the region of the scapula. P. 25mm

SI.10
Shoulder and arm weakness and aches. P. 25mm

SI.11
Pain in the rear-side of the elbow and arm, pain in the region of the scapula. O. 25mm

SI.12
Aches and numbness in head and arm, pain in the region of the scapula. P. 15mm

SI.13
Stiffness and pain in the region of the scapula. P. 12.5mm

SI.14
Neck rigidity, back and shoulder ache. O. 15mm

SI.15
Pain in back and shoulder, cough and asthma. O. 15mm

SI.16
Neck pain and rigidity, sore throat, ringing in the ears and deafness. P. 20mm

SI.17
Globus hystericum, swelling of the cheek area, ringing in the ears, deafness. P. 20mm

SI.18
Toothache, yellow sclera, paralysis of the face, twitching of eyelids. P. 20mm

SI.19
Ear discharge, ringing in the ears, deafness. P. 25mm

MAJOR LEG POINTS

STOMACH CHANNEL

ELEMENT—Earth
ORGAN—Stomach   **TYPE:** Hollow organ
HUMOR—Kapha (Primary)
TIME OF ENERGY PEAK—7-9 a.m.
CHANNEL LOCATION—Front aspect of leg.

ST.45 (WELL)—Wind
   Mental confusion, febrile diseases, dream disturbed sleep. facial swelling, nosebleed, deviation of the mouth, toothache, distending sensation of the chest and abdomen, foot and leg coldness. O. 4mm

ST.44 (SPRING)—Water
   Febrile diseases, toothache, nosebleed, deviation of the mouth, diarrhea, distention or pain in abdomen, dysentery, pain and swelling of dorsum of foot. P. 12.5mm

ST.43 (STREAM)—Ether
   Abdominal noises, facial or general swelling, abdominal pain and swelling of the foot dorsum. P. 15mm

ST.42 (SOURCE)
   Paralysis in the facial area, motor impairment and muscular atrophy of foot, swelling and redness of the foot dorsum. P. 8mm

ST.41 (RIVER)—Fire
   Depressive mental disorders, headaches, dizziness/vertigo, head and face edema, abdominal distention, constipation; muscular atrophy, motor impairment/pain and paralysis of the lower extremities. P. 15mm

ST.40 (BRIDGE POINT)
   Mental disorders, headaches, dizziness, epilepsy, asthma, sore throat, chest pain, excessive sputum; muscular atrophy, motor impairment, pain, paralysis or swelling of the lower extremities. P. 25mm

ST.39
   Pain in lower abdomen, mastitis, lower extremities pain, paralysis and motor impairment and muscular atrophy; ache in back referring to testicles. P. 25mm

ST.38
   Leg and shoulder pain/paralysis, motor impairment and muscular atrophy. P. 25mm

ST.37
   Hemiplegia, pain and distention in abdomen, noises in the abdomen, dysentery, diarrhea, appendicitis, beri-beri. P. 25mm

ST.36 (SEA)—Earth
   Mental disorders, dizziness, hemiplegia, abdominal pain and distention, stomach pain, vomiting, indigestion, diarrhea, constipation, dysentery, noises in the abdomen, mastitis, beri-beri, knee joint and leg aches. P. 25mm

ST.35
   Motor impairment, numbness and pain in knee, beri-beri. O. 25mm

ST.34
   Gastric pain, mastitis, motor impairment of the leg, swelling and pain in knee. P. 25mm

ST.33
   Leg numbness/ motor impairment and pain. P. 25mm

ST.32
   Lumbar and iliac pain, leg motor impairment and pain, coldness in knee, beri-beri. P. 25-30mm

ST.31
Leg muscular atrophy/ motor impairment, pain and numbness, thigh pain. P. 25-30mm

ST.30
Irregular menstruation, hernia, swelling and pain in external genital area. P. 25mm

ST.29
Hernia, pain in abdomen, amenorrhoea, uterine prolapse. P. 25mm

ST.28
Hernia, urine retention, distention in the lower abdominal area (Vata). P. 25mm

ST.27
Hernia, urine retention, seminal emission, distention in the lower abdominal area. P. 25mm

ST.26
Hernia, pain in abdominal area. P. 25mm

ST.25 (Large Intestine Organ Front Point)
Edema, diarrhoea, constipation, dysentery, irregular menstruation; noises, distention and pain in abdominal area.
P. 25mm

ST.24
Mental disorders, pain in the gastric region, vomiting. P. 25mm

ST.23
Mental disorders, restlessness and irritability, indigestion and pain in the gastric region. P. 25mm

ST.22
Edema, anorexia, diarrhoea, noises, distention and pain in the abdomen. P. 25mm

ST.21
Anorexia, vomiting, loose stools, pain in the gastric region. P. 25mm

ST.20
Anorexia, vomiting, distention in the abdomen, pain in the gastric region. P. 25mm

ST.19
Anorexia, vomiting, distention in the abdomen, pain in the gastric region. P. 15mm

ST.18
Asthma, mastitis, cough, chest pain, deficiency in lactation. O. 8mm

ST.17
Not to be punctured (nipple).

ST.16
Asthma, mastitis, cough, chest fullness and pain. O. 8mm

ST.15
Asthma, mastitis, cough, chest fullness and pain. O. 8mm

ST.14
Cough, hypochondria and chest pain and fullness. O. 8mm

ST.13
Asthma, cough, chest fullness. P. 8mm

ST.12
Asthma, sore throat, cough, supraclavicular fossa region pain. P. 8mm

ST.11
Asthma, sore throat P. 10mm

ST.10
Asthma, sore throat P. 12.5mm

ST.9
Dizziness, flushing of the face, asthma, sore throat. P. 12.5mm

ST.8
Headaches, eye pains, blurred vision, tears aggravated by wind. H. 25mm (along scalp)

ST.7
Toothache, jaw motor impairment, arthritis in the jaw, noises in the ear, ear discharges, facial paralysis. P. 12.5mm

ST.6
Toothache, facial paralysis, motor disturbance of the trigeminal nerve, mumps, neck stiffness and pain, swelling of the cheek area, arthritis in the jaw. P. 12.5mm

ST.5
Toothache, motor disturbance of the trigeminal nerve, swelling of the cheek area, mouth deviation, stomatitis. O. 8mm (towards ST.6)

ST.4
Imbalance in salivation, mouth deviation, twitching eyelid. O. 25mm

ST.3
Toothache, facial paralysis, twitching eyelid, nosebleed, cheek and lip swelling and pain. P. 10mm

ST.2
Pain and paralysis of the face, eye redness and pain, twitching of eyelid, myopia. P. 8mm

ST.1
Paralysis of the face, eye redness, pain, swelling, conjunctivitis, tears made worse by wind, night blindness, twitching eyelid and myopia. P. 15mm

GALLBLADDER CHANNEL

ELEMENT—Ether
ORGAN—Gallbladder   **TYPE:** Hollow Organ
HUMOR—Pitta (Secondary)
TIME OF ENERGY PEAK—11 p.m.-1 a.m.
CHANNEL LOCATION—Outside of leg.

GB.44 (WELL)—Wind
Febrile diseases, dream disturbed sleep, deafness, one-sided headache, pain in eye, pain in the hypochondria. O. 6mm

GB.43 (SPRING)—Water
Febrile diseases, headache, blurred vision, pain in outer canthus, deafness,ringing in the ears, cheek pain, submandibular, costal and hypochondria pain. O. 8mm

GB.42
Painful and red eyes, axillary swelling. foot dorsum swelling and redness, distending pain in breast. P. 10mm

GB.41 (STREAM)—Ether
Malaria, pain in outer canthus, blurred vision, costal and hypochondria pain, mastitis, foot dorsum pain and swelling. P. 12.5mm

GB.40 (SOURCE)
Malaria, neck/chest and hypochondria pain, axillary swelling, vomiting, acid regurgitation, muscular atrophy, motor impairment/ weakness and pain in lower extremities, pain and swelling of lateral aspect of ankle joint. P. 12.5mm

GB.39
Rigidity in neck area, abdominal distention, chest fullness, hemiplegia, leg/knee and hypochondria pain, beri-beri, knee and ankle arthritis. P. 12.5mm

GB.38 (RIVER) – Fire
Malaria, one-sided headache, outer canthus/supraclavicular fossa and axillary pain, scrofula, pain in chest/hypochondria and lateral aspect of lower extremities, arthritis in knee. P. 15mm

GB.37 (BRIDGE POINT)
Knee pain, muscular atrophy, motor impairment and pain in leg, eye pain, myopia, night blindness, breast pain. P. 25mm

GB.36 (CLEFT)
Neck, chest and hypochondria pain, cramp in calf. P. 20mm

GB.35
Pain in knee, hypochondria and chest fullness, foot weakness and muscular atrophy. P. 20mm

GB.34 (SEA) – Earth
Hemiplegia, bitter taste in mouth, vomiting, constipation, muscular atrophy/motor impairment/numbness and pain of the lower extremities, knee pain and swelling, hypochondria and costal pain, high blood pressure. P. 25mm

GB.33
Leg numbness, knee pain and swelling, tendon contracture in rear of the knee. P. 12.5mm

GB.32
Hemiplegia, leg muscular atrophy/ numbness/ pain, motor impairment and weakness. P. 20mm

GB.31
General itching, hemiplegia, sciatica, leg pain/motor impairment and muscular atrophy, paralysis in children, knee arthritis. P. 25mm

GB.30
Hemiplegia, hip and lower back pain, sciatica, leg pain/weakness/ motor impairment and muscular atrophy, paralysis in children. P. 25-50mm

GB.29
Leg and back paralysis and pain. P. 25mm

GB.28
Uterine prolapse, leukorrhea, pain in lower abdomen/ hip and lower back. P. 25mm

GB.27
Hernia, leukorrhea, hip and lower back pain. P. 25mm

GB.26
Hernia, leukorrhea, irregular menstruation, hypochondria and lower back pain. P. 25mm

GB.25 (Kidney Organ Front Point)
Distention in abdomen, diarrhea, abdominal noises, hypochondria and lower back pain. P. 25mm

GB.24 (Gallbladder Organ Front Point)
Jaundice, hiccup, vomiting, regurgitation. O. 12.5mm

GB.23
Asthma, chest fullness. O. 12.5mm

GB.22
Auxillary swelling, hypochondria pain. O. 12.5mm

GB.21
Apoplexy, mastitis, neck rigidity, shoulder and back pain, arm and hand motor impairment. P. 12.5mm

GB.20
Febrile diseases, headaches, common cold, dizziness, rhinorrhea, pain and redness in eyes, neck pain and stiffness, back and shoulder pain. P. 25mm

GB.19
Headaches, neck stiffness and pain. H. 12.5mm (along skin)

GB.18
Headaches, nosebleeds and rhinorrhea. H. 12.5mm (along skin)

GB.17
Headaches on one side of the head, blurred vision. H. 12.5mm (along skin)

GB.16
Headaches, painful and red eyes, blurred vision. H. 12.5mm (along skin)

GB.15
Headaches, obstructions in nasal passage, blurred vision, tears made worse by wind. H. 12.5mm (along skin)

GB.14
Frontal headaches, twitching of eyelid, blurred vision. H. 12.5mm (along skin)

GB.13
Headaches, blurred vision, epilepsy. H. 12.5mm (along skin)

GB.12
Insomnia, headaches, toothaches, facial paralysis, s/neck stiffness and pain, cheek swelling. O. 12.5mm (down)

GB.11
Headaches, earaches, deafness, ringing in the ears, neck pain. H. 8mm (along skin)

GB.10
Headaches, ringing in the ears, deafness. H. 8mm (along skin)

GB.9
Depressive mental disturbances, headaches, gum swelling. H. 8mm (along skin)

GB.8
Headaches on one side of the head (Pitta type). H. 12.5mm (along skin)

GB.7
Temporal headaches (Pitta), cheek and jaw swelling, lockjaw. H. 8mm (along skin)

GB.6
Temporal headaches (Pitta). H. 8mm (along skin)

GB.5
Temporal headaches (Pitta). H. 12.5mm (along skin)

GB.4
Temporal headaches (Pitta), blurred vision, ringing in the ears. H. 12.5mm (along skin)

GB.3
Headaches, toothache, ringing in ears, facial paralysis and deafness. P. 8mm

GB.2
Toothaches, ringing in ears, deafness, facial paralysis. P. 15mm

GB.1
Headaches, tears and red eyes, progressive loss of vision. H. 8mm (along skin)

URINARY BLADDER CHANNEL

ELEMENT — Water
ORGAN — Urinary Bladder   **TYPE:** Hollow Organ
HUMOR — Vata (Secondary)
TIME OF ENERGY PEAK — 3-5 p.m.
CHANNEL LOCATION — Rear aspect of leg, back and head.

UB.67 (WELL) — Wind
    Headache, nosebleed, nasal obstruction, pain in eyes, difficult labor, heat in sole of the foot. O. 4mm

UB.66 (SPRING) — Water
    Blurred vision, headache, neck rigidity, nosebleed. P. 6mm

UB.65 (STREAM) — Ether
    Headaches, mental confusion, neck rigidity, blurred vision, backache, pain in rear of leg. P. 8mm

UB.64 (SOURCE)
    Headaches, dizziness, epilepsy, neck rigidity, lower back and leg pain (Vata). P. 12.5mm

UB.63 (CLEFT)
    Convulsions in infants, epilepsy, backache, leg motor impairment and pain. P. 12.5mm

UB.62
    Mental confusion, insomnia, headaches, dizziness, epilepsy, leg and back aches. P. 8mm

UB.61
    Leg weakness and muscular atrophy, heel pain. P. 12.5mm

UB.60 (RIVER) — Fire
    Headache, blurred vision, nosebleed, rigidity of neck, shoulder and arm spasms and pain, backache, heel and ankle pain, epilepsy in children, difficult labor, sciatica. P. 12.5mm

UB.59
    Headache, head heaviness, pain in eye, lower back pain, leg paralysis, kidney and bladder inflammation, external malleolus swelling and redness, rheumatoid arthritis. P. 25mm

UB.58 (BRIDGE POINT)
    Headache, blurred vision, obstruction of the nasal passages. nosebleed, lumbago, leg weakness. P. 25mm

UB.57
    Hemorrhoids, constipation, leg pain, pain in lower back, rectal prolapse, beri-beri. P. 25mm

UB.56
    Hemorrhoids, acute pain in lower back, leg pain. P. 25mm

UB.55
    Backache, leg ache/ paralysis and numbness. P. 25mm

UB.54
    Hemorrhoids, lumbar-sacral pain, leg muscular atrophy/pain and motor impairment, sciatica. P. 25mm

UB.53
    Distention and noises in abdomen, lower back pain. P. 25mm

UB.52
    Impotence, seminal emission, urine retention, lower back pain/swelling and stiffness. P. 25mm

UB.51
    Constipation, epigastric pain, masses in abdomen, leg and neck pain. P. 25mm

UB.50
Distention in abdomen, epigastric and back pain. O. 12.5mm

UB.49
Difficulty in swallowing, distention in abdomen, diarrhea, noises in abdomen, vomiting, lumbago, sciatica, cystitis, hemorrhoids. O. 12.5mm

UB.48
Jaundice, diarrhea, noises in abdomen, pain in abdomen. O. 12.5mm

UB.47
Chest, back and hypochondria pain, diarrhea, vomiting. O. 12.5mm

UB.46
Vomiting, belching, back pain and stiffness, difficulty in swallowing. O. 12.5mm

UB.45-44
Asthma,cough, shoulder and back pain and stiffness. O. 12.5mm

UB.43
Poor memory, asthma, cough, lung tuberculosis, coughing up blood, night sweating, indigestion, seminal emission. O. 12.5mm

UB.42
Asthma, cough, lung tuberculosis, shoulder and back pain, rigidity in neck. O. 12.5mm

UB.41
Neck, shoulder and back pain and stiffness, elbow and arm numbness. O. 12.5mm

UB.40 (SEA)—Earth
Lower back pain, hip joint motor impairment, muscular atrophy, abdominal pain, vomiting and diarrhea. P. 25mm

UB.39
Lower back stiffness and pain, distention in the lower abdomen (Vata),leg and foot cramps, urine emission. P. 25mm

UB.38
Contracture of tendons on rear of knee, numbness in thigh. P. 25mm

UB.37
Thigh and lower back pain. P. 25mm

UB.36
Sacral and lumbar pain, hemorrhoids. P. 25mm

UB.35
Diarrhea, dysentery, impotence, leukorrhea. P. 25mm

UB.34
Lower back pain, lower abdominal pain, urine retention/difficulty, constipation. P. 25mm

UB.33
Constipation, pain in lower back, urine retention, leukorrhea, irregular menstruation, sciatica, hemorrhoids. P. 25mm

UB.32
Rheumatism, motor impairment and muscular atrophy of the leg, hernia, leukorrhea, irregular menstruation, pain in the lower back, sciatica, hemorrhoids. P. 25mm

UB.31
Uterine prolapse, irregular menstruation, urine retention, leukorrhea, pain in lower back, sciatica, hemorrhoids. P. 25mm

UB.30
Irregular menstruation, leukorrhea, seminal emission, endometriosis, sciatica, hernia, hip and lower back pain. P. 25mm

UB.29
Hernia, dysentery, lower back stiffness and pain. P. 25mm

UB.28 (Urinary Bladder Organ Rear Point)
Diarrhea, constipation, urine emission and retention, seminal emission, pain and distention in lower abdomen. P. 25mm

UB.27
Urine emission, dysentery, seminal emission, pain and distention in lower abdomen. P. 25mm

UB.26
Diarrhea, distention in abdomen, pain in lower back. P. 25mm

UB.25 (Large Intestine Organ Rear Point)
Pain and distention in abdomen, constipation, enteritis, diarrhea, noises in the abdomen, pain in lower back, paralysis in infants. P. 25mm

UB.24
Pain in lower back, lumbago, hemorrhoids. P. 25mm

UB.23 (Kidney Organ Rear Point)
Blurred vision, ringing in the ears, deafness, impotence, urine emission, leukorrhea, ache in back, knee weakness, seminal emission, irregular menstruation, nephritis. P. 25mm

UB.22 (Tridosha Rear Point)
Vomiting, indigestion, dysentery, diarrhea, noises and distention in abdomen, lower back stiffness and pain. P. 25mm

UB.21 (Stomach Organ Rear Point)
Vomiting, nausea, indigestion, noises in the abdomen, distention in abdomen, chest/epigastric and hypochondria pain. O. 12.5mm

UB.20 (Spleen Organ Rear Point)
Jaundice, diarrhea, dysentery, vomiting, indigestion, distention in abdomen, back pain and swelling. O. 12.5mm

UB.19 (Gallbladder Organ Rear Point)
Lung tuberculosis, bitter taste in mouth, jaundice, fever, chest and hypochondria pain. O. 12.5mm

UB.18 (Liver Organ Rear Point)
Mental confusion, epilepsy, blurred vision, night blindness, nosebleed, jaundice, hepatitis, redness in eye, coughing of blood, pain in the back and hypochondria. O. 12.5mm

UB.17
Cough, asthma, difficulty in swallowing, hiccup, vomiting, coughing up blood, night sweating, fever (Vata type). O. 12.5mm

UB.16
Pain in heart and abdomen(due to its location). O. 12.5mm

UB.15 (Heart Organ Rear Point)
Mental lapse, irritability, panic, epilepsy, palpitations, coughing up of blood, cough. O. 12.5mm

UB.14 (Pericardium Organ Rear Point)
Mental disturbance and restlessness, palpitations, cardiac pain, heart disease, gastric ulcer, vomiting. O. 12.5mm

UB.13 (Lung Organ Rear Point)
Asthma, common colds, bronchitis, coughing up blood, cough, night sweating, Vata type fever. O. 12.5mm

UB.12
Headache, cough, common cold, fever, backache, rigidity of neck. O. 12.5mm

UB.11
Headache, cough, fever, scapular aches, neck rigidity. O. 12.5mm

UB.10
Headaches, obstruction in nasal passage, neck, back and shoulder pain. P. 12.5mm

UB.9
Headache, obstruction in nasal passage. H. 12.5mm

UB.8
Mental confusion, ringing in the ears, dizziness. H. 12.5mm

UB.7
Headache, nosebleed, dizziness, obstruction in nasal passage. H. 12.5mm

UB.6
Headache, blurred vision, obstruction in nasal passage. H. 12.5mm

UB.5
Headache, epilepsy, blurred vision. H. 12.5mm

UB.4
Frontal headache, nosebleed, obstruction in nasal passage, blurred vision. H. 12.5mm

UB.3
Headache, epilepsy, dizziness. H. 12.5mm

UB.2
Headaches, twitching eyelid, blurred vision, eye redness/pain and swelling. H. 12.5mm

UB.1
Night blindness, color blindness, eye redness/ pain and swelling, cataract. P. 6mm

LIVER CHANNEL

ELEMENT—Ether
ORGAN—Liver   **TYPE**: Solid Organ
HUMOR—Pitta (Secondary)
TIME OF ENERGY PEAK—1-3 a.m.
CHANNEL LOCATION—Inside area of leg

Lv.1 (WELL)—Ether
Uterine prolapse and hemorrhage, hernia, urine emission. O. 6mm

Lv.2 (SPRING)—Fire
Insomnia, headache, blurred vision, glaucoma, menorrhagia, epilepsy, eye swelling/pain and redness, hernia, pain in urethra, urine retention, hernia, deviation of mouth, convulsion. O. 12.5mm

Lv.3 (STREAM)—Earth
Insomnia, headache, high blood pressure, vertigo, epilepsy, diabetes, jaundice, uterine bleeding, amenorrhea, hernia, urine retention, urine emission, deviation of mouth, convulsion in infants. P. 12.5mm

Lv.4 (RIVER)—Wind
Seminal emission, pain on outside of genitals, retention of urine, hernia. P. 12.5mm

Lv.5 (BRIDGE POINT)
Irregular menstruation, leg pain, difficulty in urination, hernia. II. 12mm

Lv.6 (CLEFT)
Uterine hemorrhage, hernia, arthritis in leg. H. 12.5mm

Lv.7
Pain in inner area of knee. P. 13mm

Lv.8 (SEA)—Water
Mania, uterine prolapse, pain in lower abdomen, difficulty urinating, pruritus in vulva, seminal emission, pain in knee/medial aspect of thigh and outside of genitals. P. 20mm

Lv.9
Irregular menstruation, difficulty in urination, pain in lumbar-sacral region and referred to lower abdomen. P. 15mm

Lv.10
Urine retention, distention in lower abdomen. P. 25mm

Lv.11
Leg and thigh pain, irregular menstruation. P. 25mm

Lv.12
External genital pain, hernia. P. 25mm

Lv.13 (Spleen Organ Front Point)
Diarrhea, vomiting, indigestion, distention in abdomen, hepatitis, costal/hypochondria and dorso-lumbar pain. P. 25mm

Lv.14 (Liver Organ Front Point)
Vomiting, hiccup, distention in abdomen, chest and hypochondria pain, chest fullness. O. 8mm

SPLEEN CHANNEL

ELEMENT—Earth
ORGAN—Spleen   **TYPE:** Solid Organ
HUMOR—Kapha (Primary)
TIME OF ENERGY PEAK—9-1 a.m.
CHANNEL LOCATION—Inner aspect of leg

Sp.1 (WELL)—Ether
Mental disorders, dream disturbed sleep, abdominal distention, uterine bleeding, convulsion. O. 4mm

Sp.2 (SPRING)—Fire
Febrile diseases without perspiration, gastric pain, abdominal distention. O. 6mm

Sp.3 (STREAM/SOURCE)—Earth
Gastric pain, abdominal distention, dysentery, vomiting, constipation, diarrhea. P. 8mm

Sp.4 (BRIDGE POINT)
Vomiting, gastric pain, abdominal noises and pain, dysentery, diarrhea. P. 25mm

Sp.5 (RIVER)—Wind
Pain and stiffness in tongue, abdominal noises and distention, constipation, diarrhea, ankle and foot pain. P. 8mm

Sp.6 (Meeting point of Spleen/Kidney/Liver channels in leg)
Insomnia, abdominal distention and noises, loose stools, irregular menstruation, uterine bleeding, leukorrhea, uterine prolapse, amenorrhea, difficult labor, seminal emission, sterility, external genital pain, hernia, difficulty in urinating, leg motor impairment and muscular atrophy/paralysis and pain. P. 25mm

Sp.7
Distention and noises in abdomen, knee and leg paralysis. P. 25mm

Sp.8 (CLEFT)
Abdominal distention, dysentery, irregular menstruation, anorexia, seminal emission and difficulty in urination. P. 25mm

Sp.9 (SEA)—Water
Abdominal distention, jaundice, diarrhea, incontinence, premature ejaculation, external genital pain, seminal emission, knee pain. P. 25mm

Sp.10
Urticaria, irregular menstruation, uterine bleeding, dysmenorrhea, amenorrhea, eczema, inner thigh pain. P. 25mm

Sp.11
Urine retention, swelling and pain in inguinal area. P. 12.5mm

Sp.12
Urine retention, hernia, pain in abdomen, endometritis, navel hernia. P. 25mm

Sp.13
Appendicitis, pain in abdomen, hernia. P. 25mm

Sp.14
Diarrhea, hernia, pain in navel. P. 25mm

Sp.15
Constipation, dysentery, indigestion, pain in abdomen. P. 25mm

Sp.16
Constipation, dysentery, indigestion, pain in abdomen. P. 25mm

Sp.17
Chest and hypochondria pain and fullness. O. 12.5mm

Sp.18
Deficiency in lactation, mastitis, cough, chest pain. O. 12.5mm

Sp.19
Chest and hypochondria pain . O. 12.5mm

Sp.20
Cough, chest and hypochondria sensation of fullness. O. 12.5mm

Sp.21 (BRIDGE POINT)
Asthma, chest pain. O. 12.5mm

KIDNEY CHANNEL

ELEMENT—Water
ORGAN—Kidney   TYPE: Solid Organ
HUMOR—Vata (Secondary)
TIME OF ENERGY PEAK—5-7 p.m.
CHANNEL LOCATION—Rear aspect of inside of leg

K.1 (Well)—Ether
Unconsciousness, pain in vertex, dizziness, blurred vision, sore throat, dryness of tongue, loss of voice, difficulty in urination, convulsion in infants, heat on the sole. P. 12.5mm

K.2 (SPRING)—Fire
Seminal emission, pruritus vulvae, uterine prolapse, irregular menstruation , coughing of blood, diarrhea. P. 8mm

K.3 (STREAM/SOURCE)—Earth
Insomnia, toothache, asthma, sore throat, deafness, coughing of blood, irregular menstruation, impotence, seminal emission, excessive urination, lower back pain. P. 8mm

K.4 (BRIDGE POINT)
Asthma, coughing of blood, difficulty in urination. P. 8mm

K.5 (CLEFT)
Blurred vision, dysmenorrhea, irregular menstruation, uterine prolapse, difficulty in urination. P. 10mm

K.6
Insomnia, epilepsy, hernia, sore throat, uterine prolapse, irregular menstruation, difficulty in urination. P. 12.5mm

K.7 (RIVER)—Wind
Night sweating, spontaneous sweating, diarrhea, abdominal distention and noises, leg muscular atrophy and swelling, foot weakness and paralysis. P. 12.5mm

K.8
Irregular menstruation, uterine bleeding and prolapse, diarrhea, constipation, pain and swelling in testicles. P. 10mm

K.9
Mental disorders, pain in medial aspect of the leg. P. 20mm

K.10 (SEA)—Water
Hernia, impotence, uterine bleeding, pain in medial aspect of thigh and knee. P. 25mm

K.11
Urine retention, impotence, external genital pain, seminal emission. P. 20mm

K.12
Leukorrhea, external genital pain, seminal emission. P. 25mm

K.13
Diarrhea, irregular menstruation. P. 25mm

K.14
Diarrhea, pain in abdomen after birth, uterine bleeding, irregular menstruation. P. 25mm

K.15
Constipation, vomiting, pain and distention in abdomen. P. 25mm

K.16
Constipation, vomiting, pain and distention in abdomen. P. 25mm

K.17
Constipation, diarrhea, distended abdomen. P. 25mm

K.18
Constipation, vomiting, pain in abdomen, pain in abdomen after birth. P. 25mm

K.19
Noises, pain and distention in abdomen. P. 25mm

K.20
Indigestion, vomiting, distention and pain in abdomen. P. 25mm

K.21
Diarrhea, vomiting, pain in abdomen. P. 15mm

K.22
Asthma, cough. O. 12.5mm

K.23
Asthma, cough, mastitis, chest and hypochondria fullness. O. 12.5mm

K.24
Asthma, cough, mastitis, chest and hypochondria fullness. O. 12.5mm

K.25
Pain in chest, cough, asthma. O. 12.5mm

K.26
Asthma, cough, chest and hypochondria fullness. O. 12.5mm

K.27
Pain in chest, cough, asthma. P. 10mm

* The flow direction of pranic energy through the channel occurs from the first point listed in each channel (well point) to the last point listed- in the case of the Kidney channel above, it is K.27, the final marma of the Kidney channel.

APPENDIX B

ACUPUNCTURE TREATMENT OF DISEASES

1. ANEMIA

Anemia is characterized by a lack of red blood cells and haemoglobin (iron carriers). It tends to reflect a lack of iron and therefore related to a vitiation of Vata. Ayurveda calls this disease Pandu Roga (pale disease).

Symptoms include paleness of the skin, especially in the inside lining of the eyelids and border of the tongue. There also tends to be low blood pressure, shallow breathing, dizziness and a rapid pulse. All of these point to a Vata derangement.

Point	Indication
L7	Dizziness
LI11	Sea point, affects Vata and the L.I.
P6	Sea point, affects and relieves the chest area (shallow breathing)
UB18	Rear Liver organ point.
UB19	Rear Gallbladder organ point.
St36	Sea point, affecting stomach, increasing Earth growth and strength in body (anti-Vata).
Sp6	Meeting point of the three solid organ channels in leg, which affect the Lower area of trunk (Vata).

2. ASTHMA

Asthma involves tightness and constriction in chest, breathing difficulties, wheezing during exhaling and is called Tomaka Shvasa in Ayurveda. Asthma attacks caused by allergens can be attributed to a lowered immune system. Ayurveda believes asthma to have gastro-intestinal imbalance origins (especially lowered Agni). Correct diagnosis is essential to ascertain which humor is vitiated. Dry wheezing cough (and triggered by nerves/stress) type relates to Vata. Phlegm congestion type involves Kapha while a rapid, rolling pulse with thick yellow tongue coating relates to Pitta.

Vata type of asthma involves needling the Lung and Large Intestine channels. This tends to eliminate Wind and coldness.

Pitta type of asthma involves needling the Sea point of the Lung channel (L5) to increase Water and decrease Fire (according to the Wheel of Control). Water controls Fire.

Kapha type asthma involves needling Stomach 40 to relax the chest and remove phlegm.

The Sea point of the Stomach channel relates to the Earth element. The Stream point of the Lung channel also relates to the Earth element. Consequently, by needling these two points (St36,L9) the Wind element (lung/L.I.) can be tonified, according to the Parent/Child concept and the Wheel of Support.

Point	Indication
Vata	
UB13	Rear Lung organ point. Balances lung.
L7	Bridge point of Lung and Large Intestine channels. Treats imbalances in these two and reduces wind and cold.
LI4	Source (Base) point of Large Intestine. Prescribed for imbalances in the large intestine (Vata's source organ).
Pitta	
St40	Bridge point of the Stomach and Spleen channels. Asthma point, removes phlegm and decreases heat in lung.
L5	Sea point (Water). Balances lung and removes heat.
Kapha	
St40	Bridge point of the Stomach and Spleen channels. Asthma point, removes phlegm.

3. AMENORRHEA

This is the imbalance involving scanty flow during menstruation. Select appropriate points of channels which are positioned in the Vata area of the trunks and the legs or of organs physically positioned in this lower trunk area (reproductive system).

Point	Indication
UB32	Removes blood stagnation in uterus.
St29	Removes blood congestion and indicated in amenorrhea.
LI4	Source (base) point of the Large Intestine channel (Vata) which affects the lower trunk.
Sp6	Meeting point of Kidney, Liver and Spleen channels. Adjusts blood flow through the reproductive system.
Lv2	Spring point, allows in and outflow of blood in liver.
Sp10	Affects the circulation of blood and promotes blood flow in menstruation.
UB18	Liver rear organ point. Affects the liver (blood flow).
UB20	Spleen rear organ point. Affects the spleen.
UB23	Kidney rear organ point. Kidney organ affects Vata and the reproductive system.
St25	Large Intestine front organ point.
St36	Sea point.

4. COMMON COLD

The common cold can be caused by four types of imbalances but essentially it is caused by a lowered immune system and is a set of symptoms which attempts to rid the body of accumulated toxins etc. The accumulation or aggravation of the three humors during a particular season and or its incorrect resolution of previous seasons (by suppressing symptoms) may lead to the common cold. The vitiation of the Tridosha or balance of the three humors may result in a chronic cold.

Point	Indications
Vata	(grey/black tongue coat/pale tongue proper)
UB12	Reduces Wind (and Vata) and alleviates headaches.
LI20	Reduces pathogenic Wind in the head area.
LI4	Source (Base) point of the L.I. increasing Fire and decreasing cold.
K7	River point increases Fire by supporting Ether (heat).
L7	Bridge point of Lung and Large Intestine channels (Vata). Relieves nasal obstruction, headaches and coughs.
Pitta	(Yellow tongue coat, red tongue proper).
GB20	Febrile diseases, common cold, headache and general Pitta head and shoulder symptoms.
3D5	Febrile diseases, headaches.
Kapha	(White tongue coat)
LI4	Source (base) point. Increases heat and decreases cold.
K7	River point. Increases Fire by supporting Ether (heat).

5. DYSMENORRHEA

Dysmenorrhea (Rakta Pradara) is a dis-function of the menstrual system and can be generally divided into two types: (a) Menorrhagia which is characterized by excessive bleeding during the monthly cycle. (b) Metrorrhagia which involves excessive bleeding at irregular intervals. Usually this is caused by an imbalance in Pitta which affects the hormones and therefore causes their imbalance. When Pitta is vitiated excess bleeding can occur anywhere in the body (e.g. rectal bleeding, nose bleeds etc.)

Point	Indication
Sp10	This point activates correct blood circulation.
Sp8	Used for pain relief during menstruation.
LI4	Used for pain relief during menstruation.

Point	Indication
St27	Removes blood stagnation and relieves pain locally in the reproductive area.
UB20/23	Regulate function of spleen and kidney (source of blood formation).
Sp6	Sea point. Strengthens spleen function (source of blood formation).
St36	Sea point. Strengthens stomach function (source of blood formation).
UB40	Sea point. Eliminates excess heat in blood (Pitta).

6. DYSENTERY

Dysentery can be of amoebic origin (pravahika) and involving Kapha or of bacillary origin (Raktatisa) and involving Pitta.

Point	Indication
Kapha	
UB20	Spleen organ point, indicated in this disorder as it warms spleen and removes intestinal congestion.
UB21	Stomach organ point, indicated in dysentery as it warms the stomach.
Sp6	This point assists in dispersing dampness (Kapha) and strengthens the function of the spleen (Kapha organ).
St36	Clears intestinal congestion.
Pitta	
St44	Spring point (Water), eliminates heat.
LI11	Sea point (Earth). Child of Fire (parent) eliminates heat, especially in the L.I.
Sp9	Sea point (Water), controls Fire (heat) by strengthening the spleen.
St25	Large intestine organ point. Indicated in dysentery by clearing congestion in the large intestine.
St37	Large intestine Sea point. Removes congestion in the large intestine.
LI4	Base (source) point of L.I. indicated in dysentery and in syndromes of the large intestine. Removes congestion in this organ.

7. DIARRHEA

Diarrhoea can be caused by an imbalance in: (1) Vata and fright (2) Pitta (3) Kapha (4) 3D (5) Treatment of Ama is best undertaken by using bitter and pungent herbs. Bitter herbs tend to dislodge the toxins (Ama) from the tissues while pungent ones consume Ama. Besides acupuncture, diarrhoea can be reduced by drinking boiled rice water (with a pinch of salt for flavor). This tends to reduce the diarrhea and is quite effective in long, drawn-out cases.

Point	Indication
St25	Large intestine organ point on front of body. Adjusts transportation and functioning of the organ proper.
UB25	Large intestine organ point on rear of body. Similarly adjusts transportation in the L.I. while also checking diarrhea.
St36	Sea point. Strengthens transportation in the spleen and stomach (Kapha).
UB23	Kidney rear organ point. Balancing kidneys to support Vata area of the trunk.
K3	Stream point (Earth). Earth (parent) supports Wind (L.I.)—(child).

8. ERYSIPELAS

Erysipelas can be caused by imbalances in: (1) Vata (2) Pitta (3) Kapha (4) 3D (5) Trauma.

Point	Indication
UB40	Sea point. Eliminates heat in the blood by acting as child, dissipating energy from parent (Fire—UB60).
P3	Sea point. Eliminates heat by encouraging Water.
LI11	Sea point .Eliminates heat from the large intestine.
LI4	Source (base) point of large intestine, eliminates heat in large intestine. Removes congestion in L.I.

9. HICCUP

Hikka Roga or hiccup is caused by vitiation of Vata. Vayu or Wind tends to rise in this case.

Point	Indication
UB17	Subdues ascending Wind (Vayu).
P6	Sea point. Affects and relieves fullness in chest area.
St36	Sea point. Indicated for treatment of stomach syndrome. Stomach is affected by rising Vayu.

10. HYSTERIA

Hysteria usually relates to Vata, the most subtle humor and one which affects the nerves.

Point	Indication
LI4	Source (base) point. Adjusts Vata by adjusting the large intestine.
Lv3	Stream point. Adjusts liver function to relieve convulsions.
K1	Well point. Subtle effect on Vata and removes unconsciousness.
P6	Stops suffocating sensations.
H7	Stream point (Earth). Indicated in hysteria. Earth tonifies Wind (child) by acting as its parent.

11. HEMORRHOIDS

Hemorrhoids (Arsha) are varicosed veins in the rectal cavity caused by congestion in the large intestine. They can be painful and can often bleed. Those that are moist and hot tend to relate to Pitta, those which are dry and painful to Vata and those which are moist and cold relate to Kapha.

Point	Indication
UB57	Indicated in hemorrhoidal syndromes.
UB32	Indicated for pain in lower back and leg.
G1	Point located in perineal area indicated for hemorrhoidal treatment due to its local position (near the rectum).

12. HIGH BLOOD PRESSURE

High blood pressure (RaktaVata) is also called hypertension. The main cause according to Ayurveda is vitiation of Vata. This then leans towards arterial hardening, narrowing and congestion (Vata can dry up moisture in blood). RaktaVata means "Vata in the blood".

Point	Indication
LI11	Sea point. Treats Wind in the large intestine and balances Vata.
St36	Sea point. This is related to Earth which is the parent of Wind. it has a tonifying effect on Vata.
GB20	Indicated for vertigo and headaches which occur in this condition.
Lv3	Stream point. Earth tonifies Wind and therefore Vata. It is indicated for vertigo and headaches.
Sp9	Sea point. As a Water point, it treats Vata by supporting the kidneys.

13. IMPOTENCE

Impotence (Klaivya) can be caused by imbalances in the following: (1) Vata (2) Pitta (3) Kapha (4) 3D It usually relates to a kidney imbalance or Vata.

Point	Indication
Vata	
UB15	Heart rear organ point. Relaxes the nervous system and therefore calms Vata.
Pitta	
H7	Stream point. This point relates to Earth which is the child of Fire
(H8).	Consequently it removes heat by sedating the Spring point.

Point	Indication
Kapha	
Sp6	This point is the junction of the Spleen, Liver and Kidney channels. They are the main protagonists in the genital and Vata area of the body.
General	
UB25	Large intestine organ rear point. Corrects Vata by affecting the large intestine.
K3	Stream point (Earth). Strengthens large intestine and Vata according to the parent/child law.

14. JAUNDICE

Jaundice (Kamala) is usually caused by the inflammation of the liver and if yellow tongue coating is found it is due to an imbalance in Pitta. Otherwise if a white tongue coating is found it is caused by vitiated Kapha affecting the liver.

Point	Indication
Kapha	
Sp9	Sea point (Water). Reduces phlegm in Kapha syndromes.
St36	Sea point (Earth). Supports the stomach in Kapha syndromes.
Pitta	
GB34	Sea point (Earth). Reduces heat or Pitta by acting as child to Fire (GB38). Affects the liver as the GB is internally related to it.
Lv3	Stream point (Earth). Reduces heat or Pitta in liver by acting as child of Fire (Lv2).
UB48	Indicated in jaundice conditions.
GB24	Gallbladder front organ point. Treatment of gallbladder syndromes, including jaundice.

15. LEUCORRHEA

Leucorrhea (Shweta Pradara), characterized by white vaginal discharge, is often caused by an imbalance in Kapha affecting the reproductive system, especially prominent in Vata females. When yellow discharge is prominent, the liver and gallbladder are also implicated.

Point	Indication
UB23	Kidney rear organ point. Tonifies Prana, especially in the kidneys (which affect the reproductive system).
UB32	this point is prescribed for leucorrhoea as it is adjacent to the affected area and in Vata channel.
UB30	As above point.
Lv5	Bridge point. This point reduces Fire and balances the liver and gallbladder.
Sp9	Sea point (Water). By tonifying this point, the spleen is strengthened, reducing heat.

16. LOW BLOOD PRESSURE

Low blood pressure (Nyuna Raktachapa) or otherwise called hypotension is normally a Vata derangement, affecting Vata constitutions.

Point	Indication
Lv3	Stream point (Earth). As the parent of Wind, Lv3 tonifies and increases the correct pranic energy levels in the L.I., to raise the blood pressure.
P6	Bridge point of 3D and pericardium, affecting flow of body fluids through the body, increasing circulation and blood pressure.

17. MALARIA

Malaria is usually triggered by the bite of a mosquito, but only in those people who are susceptible to the disease, according to Tridosha imbalances. Treatment is according to symptoms, especially fever (Pitta) and mental confusion (Vata).

Point	Indication
Pitta	
P5	River point (Wind). P5 acts as the parent of the Sea point (P3) which represents Water. By treating the parent the child is supported and increased, tending to eliminate internal heat and fever.
SI3	Stream point (Ether). Indicated in malaria and febrile conditions, dispersing heat in the external disease pathway (Pitta).
Vata	Mental confusion. Use the twelve Well points located in both arms since they deal with the most subtle (Ether) and Vata.

18. MUMPS

Mumps (Karnamulaka) are usually caused by a Pitta infection or imbalance. It is characterized by inflammation and swelling. There is yellow urine and thirst. The heat affects the large intestine and 3D channels which cross the swollen area.

Point	Indication
LI4	Source (base) point.Indicated in facial swelling by eliminating heat in the large intestine (and face) via its channel. LI11 Sea point (Earth). It drains heat from Fire as its child and thereby removing heat in the L.I.
3D17	Located in the area, it relieves swelling and pain in the affected region. St6 Located in the area, it relieves swelling and pain in the affected region.

19. PNEUMONIA

Pneumonia (Shwasanka Jwara) is usually caused by fever due to disturbance of Vata, causing inflammation in lung (a Vata organ).

Fever/Headaches

GB20, LI4, K7, H9

Cough/Chest pain

L5, L9.

Point	Indication
Others	
UB13	Lung rear organ point. Treatment of lung syndromes, especially with fevers.
LI11	Sea point (Earth). Child of Fire, removing heat in L.I.
P6	Stops suffocating sensations in chest.
3D6	River point. Used in chest disorders (Kapha area).

20. TONSILLITIS

Tonsillitis (Tundikeri) or inflammation of the tonsils is usually caused by vitiation of Pitta, affecting the lung.

Point	Indication
L10	Spring point. Reduces Fire in lung.
K3	Stream point (Earth). Reduces Fire by acting as its child. The Kidney channel runs along the throat area and thereby affecting it.
LI4	Source (base) point. Indicated for sore throat, by balancing LI and Lung channels (Vata).
L11	Indicated for sore throat, fever in lung and respiratory system.

APPENDIX C—RESOURCES

INTERNATIONAL FEDERATION OF AYURVEDA

Interest around the world has created several Ayurvedic Associations worldwide. These have now been formally united with the formation of the International Federation of Ayurveda (I.F.A.). This officially took place at the 2nd International Ayurvedic Conference in Pune, held in January 1993.

The current Head Office of the Federation is in Adelaide, Australia. For details about your local association or the Federation, please contact the International President of the I.F.A.:

Dr. Krishna Kumar,
International Federation of Ayurveda,
27 Blight Street,
Ridleyton S.A. 5008
AUSTRALIA
Telephone: (08) 346 0631

AUSTRALIAN INSTITUTE OF AYURVEDIC MEDICINE

The Australian Institute has since 1970 continued promoting Ayurveda in Australia via teaching of this most excellent art and science (Ayurveda and Ayurvedic Acupuncture).

Certificate, Diploma and Degree courses are available at the Institute for those who wish to qualify as ayurvedic physicians or who instead be interested in Ayurveda as a means of self healing. An integral part of the course is graduation in Ayurvedic Acupuncture.

Currently, the Institute is the only teaching establishment in Australia where the traditional Ayurvedic Acupuncture system can be studied.

For further information contact:

AUSTRALIAN INSTITUTE OF AYURVEDIC MEDICINE
19 Bowey Avenue
Enfield S.A. 5085
Australia
Telephone: (08) 349 7303

To study Ayurvedic medicine:

Ayurvedic Holistic Center
82A Bayville Ave.
Bayville. N.Y. 11709

Ayurvedic Living Workshops
P.O. Box 188
Exeter, Devon EX4 5AB
ENGLAND

The Ayurveda Center of Santa Fe
1807 Second St. Suite 20
Santa Fe, N.M. 87505
(505) 983-8898

Lotus Ayurvedic Center
4145 Clares Street Suite D
Capitola, CA 95010
(408) 479-1667

Maharishi Health Center
Hale Clinic
7 Park Crescent
London, W14 3H3
ENGLAND

Natural Therapeutics Center
'Surya Daya'
Gisingham, Nr. Iye
Suffolk, ENGLAND

Victoria Stern N.D.
P.O. Box 1814
Laguna Beach, CA 92652
(714) 494-8858

Correspondence Courses

American Institute of Vedic Studies
Attn. David Frawley
P.O. Box 8357
Santa Fe, N.M. 87504
(505) 983-9385

Institute for Holistic Education
33719 116th Street A.A.
Twin Lakes, Wisconsin 53181
(414) 877-9396

Lessons and Lectures in Ayurveda
by Dr. Robert Svoboda
P.O. Box 23445
Albuquerque, N.M. 87192-1445
(505) 291-9698

To receive Pancha Karma:

The Ayurveda Center of Santa Fe
1807 Second St. Suite 20
Santa Fe, N.M. 87505
(505) 983-8898

Diamond Way Health Associates
214 Girard Blvd. N.E.
Albuquerque, N.M. 87106
(505) 265-4826

Lotus Ayurvedic Center
4145 Clares Street Suite D
Capitola, CA 95010
(408) 479-1667

Maharishi Health Center
Hale Clinic
7 Park Crescent
London, W14 3H3
ENGLAND

Dr. Lobsang Rapgay
2931 Tilden Ave.
Los Angeles, CA 90064
(310) 477-3877

Victoria Stern N.D.
P.O. Box 1814
Laguna Beach, CA 92652
(714) 494-8858

**Sources for Ayurvedic Books, Products,
Herbs, Essential Oils and Supplements:**

Auroma International, Inc.
P.O. Box 1008-AA
Silver Lake, WI 53170
(414) 889-8569
(incense and essential oils)

Ayush Herbs, Inc.
10025 N.E. 4th St.
Bellevue, WA 98004
(800) 925-1371

Bazaar of India Imports, Inc.
1810 University Ave.
Berkeley, CA 94703
(510) 548-4110

Bioveda
P.O. Box 420
Conger, N.Y. 10920

Herbal Vedic Products
P.O. Box 6054-AA
Santa Fe, N.M. 87502
(herbal body care and supplements)

Lotus Fulfillment Service (retail)
33719 116th St., Dept. AA
Twin Lakes, WI 53181
(414) 889-8501
(complete range of items)

Lotus Herbs
1505 42nd Ave., Suite 19
Capitola, CA 95010
(408) 479-1667

Lotus Light Natural Body Care
    (wholesale)
P.O. Box 1008, Dept. AA
Silver Lake, WI 53170
(414) 889-8501; fax (414) 889-8591
(complete selection of over 7,000 items)

Wishing Well Video
P.O. Box 1008-AA
Silver Lake, WI 53170
(414) 889-8501
(wide range of videos on alternative
    health and healing)

BIBLIOGRAPHY

Birnbaum, Raoul. *THE HEALING BUDDHA*. Rider and Co., London 1980.

Callinan, Paul. *WHOLISTIC BODY SIGNATURES*. Australian Well-being Magazine, Vol 31.

Charaka. (Sharma R.k., and Dash B.). *CHARAKA SAMHITTA*. Chowkhamba Sanskrit Series, Varanasi, India.

Dash, Bhagwan. *AYURVEDA FOR MOTHER AND CHILD*. Delhi Diary Publishers, New Delhi 1988.

Dash, Bhagwan and Manfred Junius. *A HANDBOOK OF AYURVEDA*. Concept Publishing Co., New Delhi.

Donden, Yeshi. *HEALTH THROUGH BALANCE*. Snowlion Publishers.

ESSENTIALS OF CHINESE ACUPUNCTURE. Foreign Language Press, Beijing.

Feuerstein, Georg. *TEXTBOOK OF YOGA*. Rider and Co., London 1975.

Frawley, David. *AYURVEDIC HEALING*. Passage Press, Utah.

Frederic, Louis. *DICTIONARY OF THE MARTIAL ARTS*. Allen and Un-win Publishers.

Heyn, Birgit. *AYURVEDIC MEDICINE*. Thorsons Publishers.

Huard, P. and Wong, M. *CHINESE MEDICINE*. World University Library, London 1968.

Iyengar, B.K.S. *LIGHT ON PRANAYAMA*. Unwin Paperbacks, London.

Kulkarni, P.H. *PROBABLE LINKS BETWEEN AYURVEDA AND ACUPUNCTURE*. Institute of Indian Medicine, Pune, India.

Lad, Vasant. *AYURVEDA-THE SCIENCE OF SELF-HEALING*. Lotus Press, Twin Lakes, Wisconsin.

Lad, Vasant and David Frawley. *THE YOGA OF HERBS*. Lotus Press, Twin Lakes, Wisconsin.

Reid, H. and Michael Croucher. *THE WAY OF THE WARRIOR.* Century Publishing.

Sharma, R.K. and Bhagwan Dash. *CHARAKA SAMHITTA.* Chowkhamba Sanskrit Series. Varanasi, India 1985.

Svoboda, Robert. *PRAKRUTI— YOUR AYURVEDIC CONSTITUTION.* Geocom Publishing, New Mexico. Distributed by: Lotus Press, Twin Lakes, Wisconsin.

Thatte, D.G. *ACUPUNCTURE MARMA AND OTHER ASIAN THERAPEUTIC TECHNIQUES.* Chaukhambha Orientalia, Varanasi, India 1988.

Thorwald, Jurgen. *SCIENCE AND SECRETS OF EARLY MEDICINE.* Thames and Hudson, London.

Veltheim, John E. *ACUPUNCTURE.* Hill of Content Publishers, Australia 1985.

Wexu, Mario. *MODERN GUIDE TO EAR ACUPUNCTURE.* Aurora Press, New Mexico.

GLOSSARY OF TERMS

ACUPUNCTURE	The system of needling pressure points for therapy
ADANKAL	Pressure points and their therapies
AGNI	Digestive/metabolic biological fire
AGNI KARMA	Heat therapy. Moxibustion
AJNA CHAKRA	Pranic flywheel between eyebrows
AKASHA	Ether, space, matter, one of the Five Elements.
ALAMBA CHAKRA	The Wheel of Support of the Five Elements
ALOCHAKA PITTA	Pitta in eyes dealing with vision
AMA	Undigested substances which develop into toxins
ANAHATA CHAKRA	Pranic flywheel in heat area
ANTAR NADIS	The channels relating to the solid organs
APANA VAYU	Prana governing downward actions in the body
ASTHI	Bone. One of the seven tissues
AVALAMBAKA KAPHA	In lung and heart, giving correct lubrication in the chest.
AYURVEDA	The Science of Life. Indian traditional medicine
BAHU	Arm
BAHYA NADIS	The channels relating to the hollow organs
BHEDANA KARMA	Piercing through Therapy. Ayurvedic Acupuncture
BHUTA AGNI	The 5 biological fires in the liver
BODHAKA KAPHA	in mouth dealing with taste
BHRAJAKA PITTA	in skin, maintaining complexion
BUDDHISM	Indian religious philosophy
CHAKRAS	Energy wheels, also cycles
CHARAKA	Ancient Ayurvedic physician
DHATUS	Tissues. The 7 tissues
DHATU CHAKRA	Wheel of the Tissues—their cycle
DARSHANA	Observation, a part of diagnosis
DOSHA	Ayurvedic 3 humors or biological forces
ETHER	Space, matter, the grid of creation
GUNA	Attribute, characteristic
GUNA DVANDVA	The Two Opposites forces
IDA	A pranic channel dealing with Kapha
JALA	The element of Water
JIHVA	Tongue diagnosis
KALARI	Ancient indian martial art
KAPHA	Biological humor related to Water and Earth, phlegm (waste product)
KARNA	Ear diagnosis
KASH	To radiate. Part of the word Akasha

KLEDAKA KAPHA	In stomach dealing with first stage of digestion
KOSTHANGAS	The major organs in the body
MAMSA	Muscle, one of the seven tissues
MANIPURA CHAKRA	Pranic flywheel in navel
MARMA	Vital pressure point
MARMA ADI	Martial art system of striking pressure points
MARMA CHIKITSA	Treatment or therapies of the Marmas or pressure points
MEDA	Fat. One of the seven tissues
MAJJA	Nerve tissue or marrow
MULADHARA CHAKRA	Pranic flywheel at base of spine
MULA MARMAS	Base vital points, where Prana is retained in channel
MOXIBUSTION	Same as agni-karma (heat therapy)
NADI	An energy (Prana) channel
NADI PARIKSHA	Pulse diagnosis
NEEDLING	Acupuncture
NIRAMA	Without Ama or toxins
NIRMANA CHAKRA	Wheel Of Creation of the Five Elements
PACHAKA PITTA	In S.I. which supports the other four Pittas
PADA	Foot or leg
PANCHA BHAUTIKA	The Five Element points
PANCHA KARMA	The five types of detox therapies
PANCHA MAHABHUTAS	The Five Elements
PANCHA SRU MARMAS	The Five Element Points in the channels
PINGALA	Pranic channel relating to Pitta
PITAR/BALA	Parent/child concept of the 5 Elements
PITTA	Biological metabolic humor, bile
PRAKOPA	Aggravation of humor
PRAKRUTI	Constitution (Vata, Pitta, Kapha)
PRANA	Biological energy
PRANAYAMA	Ayurvedic and Yogic breathing system
PRANIC MANDALA	Ayurvedic Bio-rhythm Clock
PRASHAMA	Alleviation of humor
PRASHNA	Questioning (in diagnosis)
PRITHVI	The Earth element
RAKTA	Blood
RANJAKA PITTA	Pitta which colors secretions
RASA	Plasma
SADHAKA PITTA	Pitta which controls intellect
SAHASRA CHAKRA	Pranic flywheel on top of head (crown)
SAMA	Possessing Ama or toxins
SAMANA VAYU	Prana governing digestion
SAMCHAYA	Accumulation of humor
SETU MARMAS	Bridge vital points connecting hollow and solid organ channels
SHASTRA	Textbook

SHUKRA	Semen, reproductive fluid
SLESHAKA KAPHA	Kapha in synovial fluid
SPARSHANA	Palpation (in diagnosis)
SROTAS	Channels carrying gross material (e.g. blood)
SUCHI	Acupuncture needle
SUCHI VEDA	Science of Acupuncture, textbook
SUSHUMNA	Pranic channel in center of spine
SURYA	Sun, an ear point treating migraines
SUSHRUTA	Ancient Ayurvedic surgeon
SVADISTHANA CHAKRA	Pranic flywheel above sex organs
TAKSHASHILA	Ancient Ayurvedic university
TARPAKA KAPHA	Kapha in brain and heart
TEJA	The element Fire
TRIDOSHA	The three humors, the Tridosha nadi or channel, the three areas of the trunk
UDANA VATA	Prana governing energy, speech, memory
VATA	The catabolic humor, related to Wind
VAYU	Wind, carrier of Prana
VEDAS	Ancient Indian sacred scriptures
VINASHA CHAKRA	Wheel of Destruction of the elements
VINAYA CHAKRA	Wheel of Control of the elements
VISSUDHI CHAKRA	Pranic flywheel in throat area
VYANA VAYU	Prana governing movement of muscles and joints and the circulation.

INDEX

ABOUT THE AUTHOR

Dr. Frank Ros A.M.D., D.Ac. is the current director of the Australian Institute of Ayurvedic Medicine, a post which he inherited and where Ayurvedic Acupuncture is taught. He was born in Algeciras, Spain and arrived in Australia in 1964 with his family. After completing his secondary education, Frank became interested in a little-known system of martial art which originated in India, thousands of years ago. His interest in this most fascinating and effective art, called Kalari, whetted his appetite for learning the higher aspects of the system, primarily Ayurvedic Acupuncture and Medicine, which began in 1970.

He graduated in 1977 with a degree in these two related systems of Indian healing, and has since practiced, taught, researched and treated at the Australian Institute and his own clinic in the district of Enfield, South Australia.

Frank is a Life Member of the prestigious Acupuncture Society of India, a government registered organization in Rajasthan (India). He is also a prominent member of the Naturopathic Practitioners Association (Australia) and of the Australian Association of Ayurveda (a member organization of the International Federation of Ayurveda).

Besides the above, Dr. Ros is also qualified in teaching the traditional Indian martial art called Kalari, one of the most ancient and effective systems in the world. Kalari or Kalaripayat means The Path of the Field of Battle, but is more correctly translated as The Way of Self-Defence, Nature's path to higher physical and mental awareness.

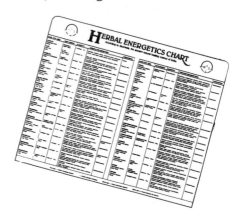

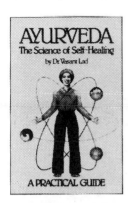

AYURVEDA

The Science of Self-Healing
A PRACTICAL GUIDE
by Dr. Vasant Lad,
Ayurvedic Physician

For the first time a book is available which clearly explains the principles and practical applications of Ayurveda, the oldest healing system in the world.

The text contains 176 well-illustrated pages which thoroughly explain the following:

History & Philosophy   First Aid
Basic Principles   Food Antidotes
Diagnostic Techniques   Medicinal Usage of
Treatment   Kitchen Herbs & Spices
Diet   And Much More

More than 50 concise charts, diagrams and tables are included, as well as a glossary and index in order to further clarify the text.

Dr. Vasant Lad, a native of India, has been a practitioner and professor of Ayurvedic Medicine for more than 20 years. He conducts the only full-time program of study on Ayurveda in the United States as Program Director of The Ayurvedic Institute in Albuquerque, New Mexico. In addition, Dr. Lad has lectured extensively throughout the U.S., and has written numerous published articles on Ayurveda.

To order your copy, send $11.95 (postpaid) to:
Lotus Press
P.O. Box 325-AA
Twin Lakes, WI 53181
Request our complete book & sidelines catalog.
Wholesale inquiries welcome.

PLANETARY HERBOLOGY

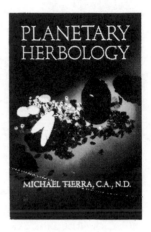

Michael Tierra, C.A., N.D.

$17.95; 485 pp.;
5½ × 8½ paper; charts.
ISBN: 0941-524272

Lotus Press is pleased to announce a new practical handbook and reference guide to the healing herbs, a landmark publication in this field. For unprecedented usefulness in practical applications, the author provides a comprehensive listing of the more than 400 medicinal herbs available in the west. They are classified according to their chemical constituents, properties and actions, indicated uses and suggested dosages. Students of eastern medical theory will find the western herbs cross-referenced to the Chinese and Ayurvedic (Indic) systems of herbal therapies. This is a useful handbook for practitioners as well as readers with a general interest in herbology.

Michael Tierra, C.A., N.D., whose very popular earlier book, *THE WAY OF HERBS,* led the way to this new major work. He is one of this country's most respected herbalists, a practitioner and teacher who has taught and lectured widely. His eclectic background studies in American Indian herbalism, the herbal system of Dr. John Christopher, and traditional oriental systems of India and China, contributes a special richness to his writing.

To order your copy, send $19.95 (postpaid) to:
Lotus Press
P.O. Box 325-AA
Twin Lakes, WI 53181
Request our complete book & sidelines catalog.
Wholesale inquiries welcome.

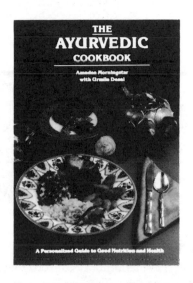

THE AYURVEDIC COOKBOOK

by Amadea Morningstar with Urmila Desai

Introduction by Dr. David Frawley

$18.95 (postpaid); 340 pp.; 6 x 9, paper; ISBN: 0-914955-06-3

The Ayurvedic Cookbook gives a fresh new perspective on this ancient art of self-healing. Over 250 taste-tested recipes specifically designed to balance each constitution, with an emphasis on simplicity, ease and sound nutrition. Designed for the Western diner, recipes range from exotic Indian meals to old American favorites. Amadea Morningstar, M.A., a Western trained nutritionist, and Urmila Desai, a superb Indian cook, are both well-versed in a variety of healing traditions. *The Ayurvedic Cookbook* includes an in-depth discussion of Ayurvedic nutrition, *tridoshic* perspectives and ways to make dietary changes that last.

"This is not just another recipe book, but a unique health manual that, if applied with proper understanding, can lead to a whole new dimension in the enhancement of health and the joy of eating."

Yogi Amrit Desai
Founder, Kripalu Center, Spiritual Director

"This book, inspired by the Ayurvedic science of nutrition, can help readers learn how to use food to enhance the quality of their lives."

Dr. Robert Svoboda, Ayurvedic physician
Author, *Prakruti, Your Ayurvedic Constitution*

"This book reveals simple recipes based upon Ayurvedic principles which can serve as a guide for an individual in his daily cooking."

Dr. Vasant Lad, Ayurvedic physician
Author, *Ayurveda, The Science of Self-Healing*
Co-author, *The Yoga of Herbs* (with Dr. David Frawley)

THE YOGA OF HERBS
An Ayurvedic Guide to
Herbal Medicine

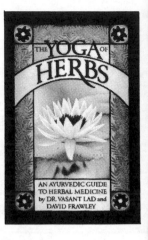

For the first time, a book is available which offers a detailed understanding and classification of herbs, utilizing the ancient system of Ayurveda. This fully developed and theoretically articulated medical system developed in India has proved itself effective for more than 5000 years as that country's classical healing tradition.

There are more than 230 herbs listed, with 88 herbs explained in detail. Included are nearly all the most commonly used western herbs according to a new and profound Ayurvedic perspective. Also a number of special powerful Ayurvedic herbs are introduced for the first time. The book is over 250 pages, with beautiful diagrams and lengthy charts, as well as a detailed glossary and index to further enhance and clarify the text.

The book combines the knowledge and experience of two respected authors in the realm of the spiritual and medical sciences of India.

Dr. Michael Tierra, Herbalist, and author of *The Way of Herbs*, says in the Foreword to this book:

> "Dr. Lad and Mr. Frawley have made a truly powerful contribution to alternative, natural health care by their creation of this important book.
>
> This book for the first time will serve not only to make Ayurvedic medicine of greater practical value to Westerners but, in fact, ultimately advance the whole system of Western herbalism forward into greater effectiveness. I think anyone interested in herbs should closely study this book whether their interests lie in Western herbology, traditional Chinese herbology or in Ayurvedic medicine."

Contents include • The Ayurvedic Theory of Herbal Medicine • How to Prepare and Use Herbs According to Ayurveda • Spiritual Usages of Herbs • How to Use Herbs According to Individual Constitutional Needs • How to Approach Western Herbs According to Ayurvedic Medical Principles • and much more.

PUBLISHED BY LOTUS PRESS
To order your copy, send $14.95 (postpaid) to:
Lotus Press
P.O. Box 325-AA
Twin Lakes, WI 53181
Request our complete book & sidelines catalog.
Wholesale inquiries welcome.